Idiotypes in Biology and Medicine

Chemical Immunology

(formerly 'Progress in Allergy')

Vol. 48

Series Editors
Kimishige Ishizaka, Baltimore, Md.
Peter J. Lachmann, Cambridge
Richard Lerner, La Jolla, Calif.
Byron H. Waksman, New York, N.Y.

KARGER

Basel · München · Paris · London · New York · New Delhi · Bangkok · Singapore · Tokyo · Sydney

Idiotypes in Biology and Medicine

Volume Editors
Dennis A. Carson, La Jolla, Calif.
Pojen P. Chen, La Jolla, Calif.
Thomas J. Kipps, La Jolla, Calif.

38 figures and 18 tables, 1990

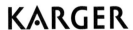

KARGER

Basel · München · Paris · London · New York · New Delhi · Bangkok · Singapore · Tokyo · Sydney

Chemical Immunology

Formerly published as 'Progress in Allergy'
Founded 1939 by *Paul Kallòs*, Helsingborg

Bibliographic Indices
    This publication is listed in bibliographic services, including Current Contents® and Index
    Medicus.

Contents

Structural Implications of AB2s.
Are Novel D Segments Involved with Anti-Idiotypic Specificity?

Patterns of Idiotypic Similarity and Their Structural Bases among
Antibodies Specific for Foreign or Self Antigens

Anti-Idiotypic Therapy of Leukemias and Lymphomas

Immunoglobulin Idiotypes in Human B Cell Neoplasia.
Implications for Pathogenesis and Therapy

Contents

Structure and Regulation of Internal Image Idiotypes

Williams, W.V. (Philadelphia, Pa.); Guy, H.R. (Bethesda, Md.); Cohen, J.A.;
Weiner, D.B.; Greene, M.I. (Philadelphia, Pa.) 185

Carson DA, Chen PP, Kipps TJ (eds): Idiotypes in Biology and Medicine.
Chem Immunol. Basel, Karger, 1990, vol 48, pp 1–13

Idiotypes and B Cell Development

John F. Kearney, Nanette Solvason, Andries Bloem, Meenal Vakil

Division of Developmental and Clinical Immunology, Department of Microbiology,
and the Comprehensive Cancer Center, University of Alabama at Birmingham, Ala.,
USA

Introduction

The network hypothesis, in its simplest form, suggests that the immune system is regulated by interactions between the variable regions of receptors found on the surface of lymphocytes [1]. While this idea has generated much interest, there is lack of direct evidence that in physiological situations immune responses are regulated in an idiotype-directed manner. However, there is now evidence that the types of interactions originally predicted do play a role in the initial establishment of the mouse B cell repertoire and that these interactions seem to occur at discrete time periods very early during development [2–4]. In fact, it has now become increasingly clear that in mouse and man the early repertoire of B cells differs considerably from that of the adult with respect to the immunoglobulin V gene expression, the specificities of Ig produced, the surface phenotype of B cells and their functions.

V Gene Usage in Early B Cells

One striking difference between the early B cell repertoire and that of the adult is the bias of the former for the expression of the most $3'$ V_H genes. Results from independent laboratories, using a variety of different methods, have demonstrated a marked preference in the early B cell repertoires in mouse originally, and now in man, for the most DJ_H proximal V_H gene families [5, 6]. Approximately 80% of hybridomas or Abelson-derived B cell lines constructed from unstimulated fetal liver and neonatal spleen express members of the V_H 7183 family, while less than 10% of B cells from normal adult spleen express V_H genes from this family. Additionally, although the V region usage of the light chains has not been analyzed, it is clear that the isoelectric focusing patterns of the immunoglobulin light chains secreted by perinatal B cell hybridomas demonstrate a limited heterogeneity when compared to those of a randomly selected panel of light chains isolated from hybridomas derived from normal adult spleens [7]. In addition, recent experiments in mice have shown that although Vκ genes do not appear to follow the paradigm provided by V_H gene usage, namely use of the most proximal genes early in development, two independent studies suggest that there is, however, a selected use of certain Vκ genes early in ontogeny [8, 9]. These results are in accord with the isoelectric focusing analysis of κ-chains used in the neonatal B cell repertoire where certain light chains were represented at a high frequency. These observations collectively provide the primary evidence that the early B cell repertoire is more restricted than the adult repertoire with respect to the expression of V_H and V_L genes.

Specificities of Antibodies from Early B Cell Repertoire

The specificities of the perinatal B cell repertoire in BALB/c mice, as determined by in vitro binding assays of hybridoma-derived monoclonal antibodies, consist of a spectrum of reactivity patterns that range from highly cross-reactive to monoreactive species. The occurrence of cross-reactive IgM antibodies decreases with the increasing age of the mice, and is rarely found in hybridomas derived from spleens of adult unimmunized mice [2–4]. Thus, the high degree of cross-reactivity is a characteristic of the early B cell repertoire. Furthermore, many of the perinatal IgM antibodies show reactivity toward idiotypic determinants on autologous immunoglobulin molecules [2, 3]. The idiotypic nature of these reactivities has been confirmed by direct binding assays using control antibodies of appropriate isotype and idiotype, as well as in classical inhibition assays where antigens (haptens as well as homologous and nonhomologous idiotypes) have been used as inhibitors. These results have been described elsewhere [2–4]. Such anti-idiotypic activity has not been detected in monoclonal antibodies secreted by hybridomas derived from spleens of normal unmanipulated or hapten-immunized adult BALB/c mice.

Functional Properties of Antibodies from the Early B Cell Repertoire

The specificity analysis of these hybridoma-derived antibodies helped identify certain monoclonal antibodies which fit into a hypothetical network shown in figure 1. BD2, a monoclonal antibody derived from liver of 2-day-old BALB/c mice, reacts with two distinct germline-encoded idiotypes, T15 and J558. These represent the major antibody idiotypes elicited in response to the antigens phosphorylcholine (PC) and $\alpha1\rightarrow3$ dextran (DEX), respectively. DB3, which reacts with BD2, is an anti-anti-idiotype antibody with respect to T15 and J558. Based on this schematic, in vivo experiments were designed to investigate the idiotype-directed activities of BD2 and DB3. Using responses to PC and DEX in adult mice as a readout system, it was shown that small doses of BD2 injected into mice at critical periods during neonatal life (5–7 days after birth for PC and 10–14 days for DEX) has a priming effect such that their immune responses to PC and DEX as adults are enhanced as compared to non-BD2-treated controls [2]. These 'developmental windows' (5–7 days for PC and 10–14 days for DEX) coincide with the first appearance of B cells capable of responding to PC and DEX, respectively, in splenic fragment cultures established with neonatal BALB/c mice as donors of precursor B cells [2]. The antibody DB3, on the other hand, when injected 1–2 days after birth leads to an enhancement of both the anti-PC and anti-DEX responses by expansion of BD2-like B cells [2].

FD5-1, shown in figure 1, is an IgG_1, κ monoclonal antibody directed toward an idiotype on the DNP-binding myeloma protein MOPC460. It was found that FD5-1 recognizes an idiotope on DB3 as well as several other DNP-binding and non-DNP-binding perinatal IgM monoclonal antibodies. FD5-1 injected in utero or into neonatal mice causes inactivation of a subset of early appearing B cells which is reflected in a failure to develop T15 and J558 idiotype-bearing B cells [3]. These observations suggest that neonatal anti-idiotype B cells may selectively expand target idiotype-bearing B cells that appear later, in a cascade-like fashion. This idea is supported by other observations described below.

In utero treatment with FD5-1 reduces the frequency of clonable IgM^+ B cells from adult spleen to two-thirds that of normal untreated controls (fig. 2). This suggests that several subsets of clonable B cells, which may normally develop, fail to do so when early appearing B cells are inactivated. These subsets do not appear to be replaced by lymphopoiesis in the adult mouse. An analysis of perinatal hybridomas producing FD5-1 reactive antibodies

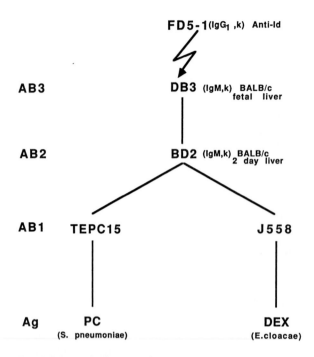

Fig. 1. Schematic diagram of interactions between hybridoma-derived immunoglobulin arranged in an AB3-AB2-AB1-Ag cascade.

showed that many of these utilize members of the V_H 7183 family. Therefore, members of this V_H gene family may confer the property to recognize and selectively expand target idiotypes upon the early B cells.

Following the identification of 'developmental windows' for the idiotypes T15 and J558, several experiments were designed to investigate the possibility that the dominance of these idiotypes was in fact due to selective expansion of B cells expressing these idiotypes [10]. Several significant findings have resulted which clearly demonstrate that interruption of the proposed mechanism alters the development of these idiotypes. The introduction of monoclonal T15+ antibodies of different isotypes between 2 and 4 days blocks the emergence of the endogenous dominant clones by apparently interfering with the interaction between the endogenous anti-T15 and T15+ B cells. Similarly, J558+ antibodies injected between 8 and 10 days after birth block the development of the endogenous J558+ B cells. Interestingly, T15 injected at 8–10 days and J558 injected 2–4 days after birth can inhibit the

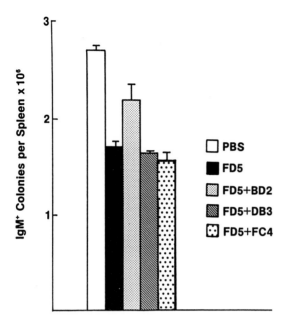

Fig. 2. This diagram describes absolute numbers of clonable B cells derived from spleens of adult mice which had been treated by transplacental transmission in utero of FD5-1 anti-idiotype antibody (solid column) compared to the number of colonies from saline-treated mice (open column). Such treatment reduces clonable B cells by one-third. As can be seen, treatment of the FD5-1-treated mice at 2 days of age with 10 μg of BD2, DB3 and FC4 did not restore the number of clonable B cells except for BD2 to some extent. This treatment as described in Vakil et al. [3] did, however, restore anti-PC responses.

reciprocal idiotype from developing normally. This suggests that a common anti-idiotypic B cell, such as one represented by hybridoma BD2, regulates the selection of both T15 and J558 idiotype clones.

A more important finding is that introduction of antigen within the first 2 days of neonatal life, in the form of the bacterial vaccine R36a or soluble polysaccharide, produces a dramatic increase in the anti-PC response of these mice when they are adults but the antibodies produced lack the normally dominant T15 idiotype [11]. An associated and potentially significant finding is that in mice primed with R36a at birth, the idiotypically linked anti-DEX response is almost totally ablated. Results from all of the experiments described above are summarized in table 1 and demonstrate functional idiotypic connectivity in mouse B cell repertoires as predicted

Table 1. Summary of the effects of various manipulations during the perinatal period on subsequent antibody responses to DEX and PC

Treatment	Age of treatment, days	Anti-PC response	T15 Id	Anti-DEX response	J558 ID
R36a (ag)	2	10-fold increase	absent	absent	absent
Dextran (ag)	7	+	+	5- to 7-fold increase	suppressed
T15 (Homologus id)	2–4	+	suppressed	+	+
T15	8–10	+	+	+	suppressed
J558	2–4	+	suppressed	+	+
J558	8–10	+	+	reduced	suppressed
BD2	5–7	3-to 4-fold increase	+	+	+
BD2	10–14	+	+	3-fold increase	+
DB3	2	2- to 3-fold increase	+	2- to 3-fold increase	+
FD5	2–4	suppressed	suppressed	+	suppressed
FD5	9–15	+	+	suppressed	suppressed

Antibody responses to PC and DEX in manipulated and control mice were analyzed following appropriate antigen challenge at 6–8 weeks of age.

+ = Antibody responses to the respective antigens in experimental mice were equivalent to those in untreated control mice.

from figure 1. These sets of experiments collectively lend support to the hypothesis that dominant clones, such as T15 and J558, are selectively expanded, not by antigen, but, by anti-idiotypic B cells during ontogeny and suggest that such mechanisms have evolved perhaps to ensure expansion of those B cell clones that offer optimal protective immunity against pathogenic bacterial infections.

IgM Antibodies Derived from Perinatal B Cell Hybridomas Are Mitogenic for Mouse B Cells

Most studies of immunoglobulins have been directed to analysis of antigen-induced antibodies and the nominal antigen-binding site. Little is known of the specificity and function of natural IgM antibodies or whether V regions of antibody molecules have functions other than binding nominal antigen through the complementarity-determining regions. It has recently been shown that there is a remarkable conservation of nucleotide sequences (amino acid residues 6–24) in framework I and (residues 67–85) in framework III between human and mouse V_H regions [12, 13]. This observation has permitted the grouping of V_H sequences into clans based on sequence homology in these regions. These particular residues are within the solvent-exposed portion of V regions, 90° away from the nominal binding site. Although there is, as yet, no evidence available, we propose that these conserved sites play a functional role other than in nominal antigen binding, and are possibly involved in the mitogenic activities observed for some neonatally derived antibodies and associated idiotype-directed interactions during B cell ontogeny.

Earlier studies performed by Coutinho et al. [14] showed that selected polyclonal and monoclonal anti-idiotypic antibodies, directed against antibodies specific for thymus-independent antigens, induced an in vitro polyclonal B cell stimulation. Certain IgM antibodies with defined idiotypic specificities can function as polyclonal activators for B cells. Apart from the relation between mitogenicity and idiotypic specificity, as defined by binding to other Ig molecules in ELISA systems, the mitogenic monoclonal IgM antibodies also seem to recognize non-Ig structure(s) expressed on a subpopulation of B cells. Initial phenotypic analysis showed a preferential binding of mitogenic IgM antibody to CD5+ B cells. A functional involvement of CD5+ B cells in these mitogenic responses was also suggested from experiments in which splenic cells from xid mice, which lack CD5+ B cells, failed to respond

Table 2. Percent positive lymphocytes

	IgM	Thy1	CD5/μ	CD8/μ
Liver	4.5	0.1	86.0	0
Spleen	23.0	0.45	67.0	0.05

Analysis for expression of Thy1- and IgM-positive cells that express CD5 or CD8 of liver and spleen cells pooled from 1- to 3-day-old mice. The frequencies were determined by microscopic examination.

to these antibodies. It is possible that the mitogenic IgM antibodies are encoded by germline genes, are expressed early in ontogeny, and are involved in the selection and expansion of the B cell repertoire during development.

Surface Phenotype of Early B Cells

CD5+ B Cells

The question then arises, are the interactions described and discussed in the previous section mediated by a subset of early appearing B cells whose immunoglobulin products use particular V region genes and express specificities which enable them to promote the development of appropriately connected B cell clones? As seen in table 2, large percentages of early B cells express the CD5 differentiation marker.

The CD5+ B cell subset predominates early in development but becomes a minor population in the adult, confined mainly to the peritoneal lymphoid population. This subset of B cells has been indirectly implicated as the B cell population responsible for the high degree of autoreactivity appearing early in development and maintained, to a lesser degree, in the adult and more directly as the B cells producing autoantibodies in man and certain autoimmune strains of mice [15–18]. Mouse CD5+ B cells express a number of properties distinct from conventional B cells: (1) they express a characteristic T cell marker (CD5) [19]; (2) when isolated from the peritoneal cavity they express MAC-1, a macrophage marker [20]; (3) they express large amounts of surface IgM and low IgD [21]; (4) they appear to have autonomous proliferative capacity and a long life span [22]; (5) they do not appear to express a hypermutation mechanism characteristic of CD5⁻ antigen-responsive B cells [22]; (6) there is some evidence that these CD5+ B cells do not appear to be derived from adult bone marrow [23]; (7) they appear to be involved in B cell lymphoproliferative diseases [24]; (8) mice which lack the CD5[+] B cell subset, such as CBA/N, are deficient in their ability to mount germline-encoded anti-polysaccharide responses [25] and have severely depressed levels of lambda light chain expression [Gollahon, pers. comm.]. All of these observations have been interpreted to suggest that CD5[+] B cells constitute a functionally distinct, and perhaps lineage-distinct, B cell subset.

Another interesting feature of CD5[+] B cells is that they appear to be the source of large amounts of IgM in the serum of unimmunized mice [26]. Additionally, mice kept in germfree environments and fed only amino acid diets maintain essentially normal levels of serum IgM. Thus, these IgM antibodies have been named 'natural antibodies' because they are present even in the absence of antigen [27]. So far, it is not clear what function these antibodies serve; although it is peculiar that the CD5[+] B cell subset appears to be responsible for their production they do not appear to participate in immune responses to a variety of T dependent antigens tested.

Because of the apparent inability of adult bone marrow to reconstitute the CD5[+] B cell subset, we have recently investigated alternative sources for their ability to reconstitute subpopulations of lymphocytes, in particular the CD5[+] B cells. In the early 1970s the omentum was shown to contain follicular aggregates of lymphoid cells which were involved in antibody production and had the ability to self-regenerate lymphocytes in diffusion chambers following supralethal irradiation [28, 29]. The omentum in the developing mouse embryo becomes distinct from the splenic and pancreatic rudiments in the mouse embryos at day 13 of gestation. At this stage it consists of a loose mesothelial sheet representing the omental primordium. Transplantation of 13-day gestation fetal omental anlage into the anterior eye chamber of a receptive host demonstrated that this tissue contains lymphoid precursors as large numbers of Thyl[+] cells and small but consistent numbers of CD5[+] cells were isolated from the graft 7 days after transplantation. Histological examination confirmed that these cells were lymphoid and of donor origin, but there was no surface or cytoplasmic immunoglobulin present and no additional staining with other lineage-specific markers which identified these lymphocytes as B and/or T cells [30].

We have repeated these experiments with some modifications to determine whether the fetal omentum might be a source of CD5[+] B cells. Our preliminary results suggest that the 13-day gestation fetal omenta as well as

Table 3. Presence of donor-derived B[1] and T[2] cells from SCID mice which received kidney subcapsular grafts of fetal primordia[3]

Graft	Spleen		PEC[4]		Lymph node		Thymus		Bone marrow	
	B	T	B	T	B	T	B	T	B	T
Liver[5]	+(<1%)[6]	+	+(42%)	+	+(<1%)	+	−	+	+	−
Omentum	+(<1%)	−	+(40%)	−	+(<1%)	−	−	−	−	−
Spleen	−	−	−	−	−	−	−	−	−	−
Bone	−	−	−	−	−	−	−	−	−	−

[1]Donor (BALB/cxC57B1/6)F$_1$ derived B cells were identified by staining first with anti-IgM FITC followed by biotinylated anti-H2D^b (detects C57B1/6 H2D) then streptavidin PE.

[2]Donor-derived T cells were identified by staining first with anti-Thy-1 FITC, followed by biotinylated anti-H2D^b then streptavidin PE.

[3]Thirteen-day gestation fetal tissues were transplanted under the kidney capsule of unirradiated SCID host.

[4]Peritoneal exudate cells.

[5]Primordia transplanted.

[6]Percent of total donor-derived B cells which are CD5$^+$.

the 13-day fetal liver, in fact, contain precursors which can give rise to CD5$^+$ B cells when transplanted under the kidney capsule of unirradiated SCID mice. However, transplantation of 13-day gestational spleen, bone or thymus under the same conditions does not give rise to this subset of B cells (table 3).

These results suggest that the CD5$^+$ B cells are a separate lineage of B cells which can be reconstituted from the mesodermally derived fetal omentum and that they migrate into sites of conventional B cell lymphopoiesis and lymphoid organization early in ontogeny. Although it is clear that in the normal adult the bone marrow may be the sole source of stem cells, the primitive mesenchymal cells in the 13-day omentum may act as an alternative source which seeds out lymphocytes early in development but later assumes a secondary role to the bone marrow. Thus, it is possible that the experimental transplantation of 13-day fetal omental tissue permits a recapitulation of these early B cell differentiation events, thereby leading to the production of CD5$^+$ B cells.

It is possible that these early B cells, by their inherent affinity for self antigens, are essential in initiating the connectivity between non-CD5⁺ B cells. The CD5⁺ B cells later, as the repertoire is established, regress to a minor subpopulation in the spleen and make up about one-half of the B cells found in the peritoneal cavity. Their role in the adult may be to maintain homeostasis of the B cell repertoire by monitoring and/or directing the repertoire using the natural IgM antibodies secreted by CD5⁺ B cells or by direct cell-cell interactions.

It is of crucial importance to dissect the elements that are necessary to reconstitute and maintain a normal functioning immune system. The role of CD5⁺ B cells very early in development may be to ensure that certain dominant clones which have the greatest protection against infection are established. It is possible that the CD5⁺ B cells are required as 'superorganizers' initially, and without their presence the normal immune repertoire does not successfully defend itself against infection.

References

1   Jerne, N.K.: Towards a network theory of the immune system. Ann. Immunol., Paris *125:* 373 (1974).
2   Vakil, M.; Kearney, J.F.: Functional characterization of monoclonal autoanti-idiotype antibodies from the early B cell repertoire of BALB/c mice. Eur. J. Immunol. *16:* 1151 (1986).
3   Vakil, M.; Sauter, H.; Paige, C.; Kearney, J.F.: In vivo suppression of perinatal multispecific B cells results in a distortion of the adult B cell repertoire. Eur. J. Immunol. *16:* 1159 (1986).
4   Vakil, M., Kearney, J.F.: Expression of idiotypes and anti-idiotypes during development: frequencies and functional significance in the acquisition of the adult B cell repertoire; in Bona, Elicitation and use of anti-idiotype antibodies and their biological properties, p. 75 (CRC Press, Boca Raton 1988).
5   Yancopoulos, G.D.; Desiderio, S.V.; Paskind, M.; Kearney, J.F.; Baltimore, D.; Alt, F.N.: Preferential utilization of the most J_H-proximal gene segments in pre-B cell lines. Nature *311:* 727 (1984).
6   Perlmutter, R.M.; Kearney, J.F.; Chang, S.P.; Hood, L.E.: Developmentally controlled expression of immunoglobulin V_H genes. Science *227:* 597 (1985).
7   LeJeune, J.M.; Briles, D.E.; Lawton, A.R.; Kearney, J.F.: Estimate of the light chain repertoire of fetal and adult BALB/cJ and CBA/J mice. J. Immun. *129:* 673 (1982).
8   Lawler, A.M.; Kearney, J.F.; Kuehl, M.; Gearhart, P.J.: Early rearrangements of early immunoglobulin κ genes unlike heavy genes show no positional bias (Submitted).
9   Kaushik, A.; Schulze, D.H.; Bona, C.; Kelsoe, G.: Murine Vκ gene expression does not follow the V_H paradigm. J. exp. Med. (In press).

10   Vakil, M.; Kearney, J.F.: Inhibition of development of T15 and J558 idiotypes by
     neonatal exposure to homologous and non-idiotypically connected antibodies in
     BALB/c mice (Submitted).

11   Vakil, M.; Kearney, J.F.: Inhibition of development of T15 and J558 idiotypes by
     neonatal exposure to phosphorylcholine and α1–3 dextran (Submitted).

12   Schroeder, H.W., Jr.; Hillson, J.L.; Perlmutter, R.M.: Early restriction of the human
     antibody repertoire. Science 238: 791 (1988).

13   Permutter, R.M.; Schroeder, H.W., Jr.; Hillson, J.L.: Diversification of the human
     fetal antibody repertoire. In Witte, Howard, Klinman, UCLA symposia on molecu-
     lar and cellular biology, New Series, vol. 85, p. 91 (Liss, New York 1988).

14   Coutinho, A.; Forni, L.; Bernabe, R.R.: The polyclonal expression of immunoglobu-
     lin variable region determinants on the membrane of B cells and their precursors; in
     Miescher, Muller-Eberhard, Springer Seminars in Immunopathology, pp. 171–121
     (Springer, Heidelberg 1980).

15   Hardy, R.R.; Hayakawa, K.; Shimizu, M.; Yamasaki, K.; Kishimoto, T.: Rheuma-
     toid factor secretion from human Leu-1+ B cells. Science 236: 81 (1987).

16   Hayakawa, K.; Hardy, R.R.; Hondo, M.; Herzenberg, L.A.; Steinberg, A.D.; Herzen-
     berg, L.A.: Ly-1 B cells: Functionally distinct lymphocytes that secrete IgM autoanti-
     bodies. Proc. natn. Acad. Sci. USA 81: 2494 (1984).

17   Manny, N.; Datta, S.K.; Schwartz, R.S.: Synthesis of IgM by cells of NZB and SWR
     mice and their crosses. J. Immun. 122: 1220 (1979).

18   Plater-Zyberk, C.; Maini, R.N.; Lam, K.; Kennedy, T.T.; Janossy, G.: A rheumatoid
     arthritis B cell subset expresses a phenotype similar to that in chronic lymphocyte
     leukemia. Arthritis Rheum. 28: 971 (1985).

19   Manohar, V.; Brown, E.; Leiserson, W.M.; Chused, T.M.: Expression of Lyt-1 by a
     subset of B lymphocytes. J. Immun. 129: 532 (1982).

20   Hardy, R.R.; Hayakawa, K.: Development and physiology of Ly-1 B and its human
     homologue Leu-1 B. A. Immunol. Rev. 93: 53 (1988).

21   Hayakawa, K.; Hardy, R.R.; Parks, D.R.; Herzenberg, L.A.: The 'Ly-1 B' cell
     subpopulation in normal, immunodefective, and autoimmune mice. J. exp. Med.
     157: 202 (1983).

22   Förster, I.; Rajewsky, K.: Expansion and functional activity of Ly-1+ B cells upon
     transfer of peritoneal cells into allotype-congenic, newborn mice. Eur. J. Immunol.
     17: 521 (1987).

23   Hayakawa, K.; Hardy, R.R.; Herzenberg, L.A.: Progenitors for Ly-1 B cells are
     distinct from progenitors for other B cells. J. exp. Med. 161: 1554 (1985).

24   Lanier, L.L.; Warner, N.L.; Ledbetter, J.A.; Herzenberg, L.A.: Expression of Lyt-1
     antigen on certain B cell lymphomas. J. exp. Med. 153: 998 (1981).

25   Martinez, A.C.; Pereira, P.; Torbio, M.L.; Marcos, M.A.R.; Bandeira, A.; De La
     Hera, A.; Marquez, C.; Cazenave, P-A.; Coutino, A.: The participation of B cells and
     antibodies in the selection and maintenance of T cell repertoires. Immunol. Rev.
     101: 191 (1988).

26   Herzenberg, L.A.; Stall, A.; Lalor, P.A.; Sidman, C.; Moore, W.A.; Parkes, D.R.;
     Herzenberg, L.A.: The Ly-1 B lineage. Immunol. Rev. 93: 81 (1986).

27   Benner, R.; Rijnbeck, A.; Bernabe, R.; Martinez, A.C.; Coutinho, A.: Frequencies of
     background Ig-secreting cells in mice as a function of organ, age and immune status.
     Immunobiology 58: 225 (1981).

28   Dux, K.; Janik, P.; Szavriawska, B.: Kinetics of proliferation cell differentiation and

IgM secretion in the omental lymphoid organ of B10/Sn mice following intra-peritoneal immunization with sheep erythrocytes. Cell. Immunol. *32:* 97 (1977).

29 Holub, M.; Hadju, I.; Trebichavsky, I.; Jaroskova, L.: Formation of lymphoid cells from local precursors in irradiated mouse omenta. Eur. J. Immunol. *1:* 465 (1971).

30 Kubai, L.; Auerbach, R.: A new source of embryonic lymphocytes in the mouse. Nature *301:* 154 (1983).

John F. Kearney, MD, 263 Tumor Institute, University of Alabama at Birmingham, University Station, Birmingham, AL 35294 (USA)

Carson DA, Chen PP, Kipps TJ (eds): Idiotypes in Biology and Medicine.
Chem Immunol. Basel, Karger, 1990, vol 48, pp 14–29

Genetic and Structural Basis of Idiotype Network

The 'GAT' Model

Michel Fougereau[a], Sylvie Corbet[a], Gilbert Mazza[a], Clara Nahmias[b], Claudine Schiff[a]

[a]Centre d'Immunologie INSERM-CNRS de Marseille-Luminy, Marseille, France;
[b]Institut Pasteur, Département de biotechnologie, Paris, France

Introduction

The idiotypic network, originally defined in a formal way by Jerne [1974], is frequently reduced to a simple cascade, written:

Ag → Ab1 → Ab2 → Ab3...,

in which Ag is the original ('external' or 'foreign') antigen, inducing the production of Ab1 or idiotype. The idiotype may induce Ab2, or anti-idiotypic antibodies, that were more recently classified into Ab2-α, or true anti-idiotypic set and Ab2-β, containing the internal image of the original antigen [Jerne et al., 1982]. This concept of an internal image is derived from the possibility of inducing Ab3 that resemble Ab1, as reported by Urbain et al. [1977] and Cazenave [1977]. From a strictly formal point of view, and as stressed by Schnurr [1981], 4 discrete types of Ab3 molecules may be anticipated: Id^-Ag^- (including antibodies directed against idiotypic specificities of Ab2), Id^+Ag^-, Id^-Ag^+ and Id^+Ag^+. The latter category is very similar, if not identical, to Ab1 and is generally referred to as Ab1'.

We have extensively analyzed the idiotypic cascade initiated by the injection in mice of the $(Glu^{60} Ala^{30} Tyr^{10})n$ random terpolymer, or 'GAT'. Most mouse anti-GAT antibodies, or Ab1, express a common set of public idiotypic specificities, termed 'pGAT', identified by a rabbit antiserum ₗThèze and Moreau, 1978], rendered idiotype specific upon appropriate absorptions.

Hybridomas derived from Balb/c mice were successfully produced at each step, Ab1, Ab2 and Ab3 [Sommé et al., 1983; Roth et al., 1985a, b] of the 'GAT' cascade and provided a source that allowed us to determine RNA nucleotide sequences of both the VH and the VL regions of the corresponding antibodies [Rocca-Serra et al., 1983a, b; Ollier et al., 1985; Roth et al., 1985a, b]. From a cDNA library, constructed from Ab1 H and L mRNA, specific VH and VL probes were derived that were used to isolate the corresponding germline genes [Schiff et al., 1986; Corbet et al., 1987].

As hybridomas were also produced in the C57 BL/6 strain, at the Ab1 [Ju et al., 1979] and the Ab3 [Roth et al., 1985a, b] levels, sequence analyses of the H and L chains were performed on mRNAs, thus providing an additional tool to approach the genetic and structural basis for idiotypy in the GAT cascade.

The Genetic Basis for the GAT Idiotypic Cascade

In the BALB/c Strain
The Ab1 and Ab3/Ab1' Are Encoded by the Same VH and Vκ Genes. A first line of evidence that mAb1s might be encoded by the same VH germline gene was derived from mRNA sequencing of four mAb1 expressing the pGAT specificities [Rocca-Serra et al., 1983b]. As two of these VH were found to be identical, it was anticipated that they might have been germline encoded. On these grounds, a specific VH cDNA probe was constructed [Schiff et al., 1983]. leading to the isolation of 3 germline genes termed H10, H4a-3 and H2b-3, 95% homologous between each other, and pertaining to the J558 family.

Interestingly, one of these 3 genes, H10, was used straightforward in the 2 VH sequences that were found to be identical. Two other Ab1 VH were clearly also derived from the same H10 gene, from which they differed only by a few somatic mutations (fig. 1). In the same figure are shown all the nucleotide sequences of 6 Ab3 antibodies that expressed the pGAT specificities, as do the Ab1. However, it is worth noting that among these 6 Ab3/Id⁺ antibodies, 4 were GAT specific, whereas 2 (namely 22.8 and 22.176) did not recognize GAT. This implies therefore that the GAT recognition is supported by a CDR which does not belong to the section encoded by a VH gene. One may also notice that Ab3 sequences are even more conserved than those

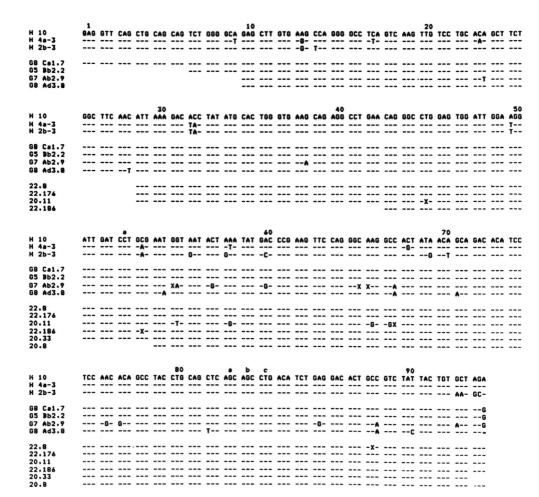

Fig. 1. The H10 germline gene encodes VH-GAT Ab1 (G series) and Ab1′ (20 and 22 series) antibodies. H4a-3 and H2b-3 are related germline genes of the J558 family. Reproduced from Schiff et al. [1986].

of Ab1s. This low level of somatic mutations may be the result of several factors: (i) fusions were made with lymphocytes derived from one single immunization, and most, but not all, chains are of the μ type; (ii) alternatively, the system may be driven by an Ig-Ig interaction (Ab1-Ab2) which is favored by germline-encoded structures. The J regions are mostly JH4 in the germline configuration. As the D region deserves some particular comments

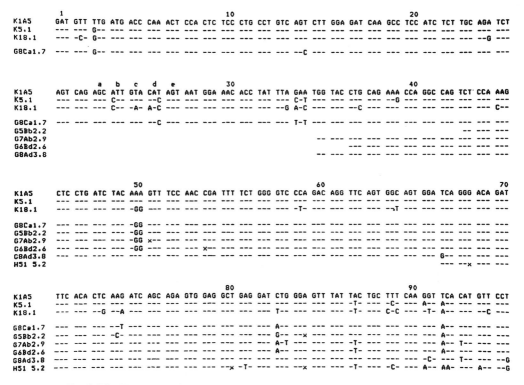

Fig. 2. The K1A5 germline gene encodes the V–GAT Ab1 antibodies. Reproduced from Corbet et al. [1987].

related to the structure-function relationship, we will return later to this problem.

Similar approaches and conclusions were made when looking at the light chain structure of Ab1/Ab3 antibodies. Three closely related genes were isolated using a 'GAT-specific' cDNA probe [Corbet et al., 1987]. These highly homologous genes constituted subgroup I of mouse κ-chains. Two of them, K1A5 and K5.1 encoded Ab1 (fig. 2) and Ab3/Id+, respectively. Again, it can be seen that light chain sequences of the Ab3/Id+ were more conserved than those of the Ab1 set, and that identical light chains were used in all Id+ antibodies, either of the Ag-Id+ or Ag+Id+ (Ab1′) type. It would thus be that the expression of the pGAT specificities are mostly dependent on the expression of VH10 and VK1.A5/VK5.1 germline genes, which would strongly suggest that this network might be germline in nature.

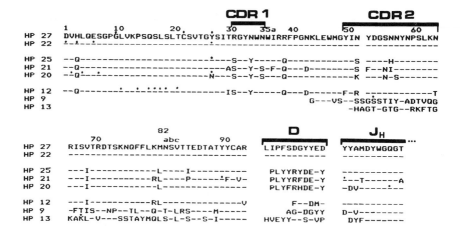

Fig. 3. Heavy chain variable region amino acid sequences derived from mRNA sequencing of Ab2 anti-idiotypes of the GAT system. Reproduced from Ollier et al. [1985].

The Ab2 and the Problem of the Internal Image. Ab2 hybridomas were prepared by immunization with polyclonal Ab1, a procedure that favors production of anti-idiotypic antibodies that are directed against the public pGAT idiotypes [Sommé et al., 1983]. Two groups of Ab2 were obtained: group 20 (HP 20, 21, 24, 25) and group 22 (HP 22, 27, 29) on the basis of discrete idiotype recognition. Antibodies of group 20 recognized part of the pGAT idiotypic mosaic that was present in all strains of mice. Antibodies of group 22 identified idiotypes mostly present in BALB/c mice.

Sequence data were obtained for H and L mRNAs of both groups. It can be seen that sequences are clearly group specific, with a remarkable conservation of H and L chain structures, within each group (fig. 3, 4), suggesting that 1 VH and 1 VL encodes the respective chains in each group, 20 and 22. Ultimate proof was not found at this level, since the germline genes were not isolated, but the conserved pattern in expressed antibodies argues strongly in favor of a germline expression at this level, which points to the existence of an idiotypic network that might be entirely germline encoded. This situation may produce an important regulatory process that might be of crucial importance in the emergence of the repertoire expressed by a highly connected set of B cells [Fougereau and Schiff, 1988]. Another strong argument in favor of a germline expression of the Ab2 level is the remarkable conservation of the D regions within each group, 20 and 22.

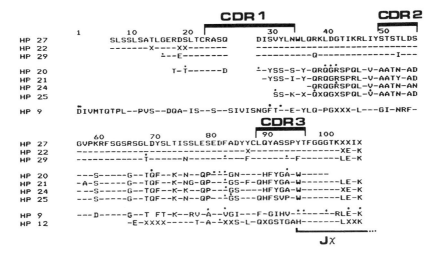

Fig. 4. Light chain variable region amino acid sequences derived from mRNA sequencing of Ab2 anti-idiotypes of the GAT system. Reproduced from Ollier et al. [1985].

Finally, a special feature was observed in these D regions, in that stretches reading *Tyr-Tyr-Glu* or *Glu-Glu-Tyr* were identified in groups 20 and 22, respectively. Since the dominant epitope of GAT is essentially composed of Glu and Tyr residues, this observation suggests that these tripeptides contained in the D region might represent the internal images of the GAT antigen.

In the C57BL/6 Strain

As already stated, the C57BL/6 mice anti-GAT Ab1 also express the pGAT specificities, identified with the xenogeneic reagent (rabbit anti-BALB/c Ab1). The same general structure should therefore be expected to be expressed in both strains, although the idiotypic mosaic is not exactly the same since there is a differential recognition by BALB/c Ab2 of group 20 and group 22, the latter being more specific of a BALB/c Ab1. Surprisingly, analysis of C57BL/6 Ab1/Ab3 VH and VL regions revealed that they differed extensively from the BALB/c sequences, the VH regions being only 75% homologous, and the Vκ 80–87% homologous between anti-GAT (or Ab3/Ab1′) of the 2 strains, as shown in figures 5 and 6. It was observed that amino acid differences were scattered all along the Vκ regions. The VH sequences

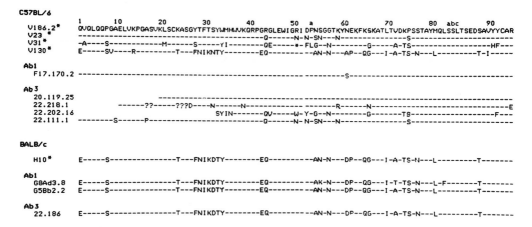

Fig. 5. Comparison of various Ab1 and Ab3 VH regions from BALB/c and C57 BL/6 antibodies with the corresponding germline genes (H10 for BALB/c and V186.2 for C57 BL/6). Taken from Corbet et al. [1988].

represented a somewhat different situation in that many of the differences, but not all, were found in CDR1 and CDR2. As hypervariable regions are most likely involved in the expression of the idiotypes, which have been shown in this case to be closely associated with the combining site, this observation leads to the conclusion that the structural basis for the pGAT idiotopes is largely degenerated. In other words, different primary structures may generate similar three-dimensional idiotopes – or more generally epitopes – that can be equally recognized by the same anti-idiotypic antiserum. This observation must be kept in mind when trying to correlate the expression of idiotypes with primary structure of immunoglobulin chains.

Allogeneic Manipulation of the GAT Idiotypic Cascade

Another intriguing observation was made regarding the usage of the BALB/c and C57BL/6 'GAT' specific VH genes. In both strains it turned out that these genes were also used in anti-NP antibodies, in association with a different D region, and with a different light chain [Rocca-Serra et al., 1983a]. The idiotypic situation for the NP system differs noticeably from that described for the pGAT idiotopes in that each strain, BALB/c and C57BL/6, expresses a different idiotype, termed NPa and NPb, respectively. Expression of NPa and NPb correlates with the discrete use of the VH genes, which are H10 and V186.2 [Bothwell et al., 1981], respectively. Allogeneic manipu-

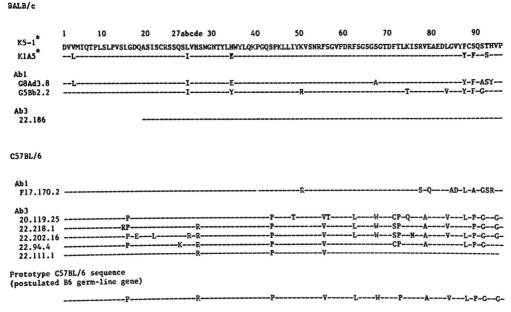

Fig. 6. Comparison of various Ab1 and Ab3 Vκ regions from BALB/c and C57 BL/6 antibodies with the major Vκ5.1 and Vκ1A5 germline genes. Taken from Corbet et al. [1988].

lation of the NP system has been attempted by Takemori et al. [1982], using various mouse strains and one (C57BL/6 × BALB/c) F1 hybrid. In BALB/c, the manipulation by Ab2 never resulted in the production of the NPb idiotype, whereas the F1 hybrid produced NPb that was exclusively of the B6 allotype. The authors concluded that this was best explained on the basis of a hole in the repertoire, the potentially 'NPb equivalent' in BALB/c [Loh et al., 1983] being presumably nonfunctional at least for this system. There was no similar attempt to produce NPa idiotype by allogeneic Ab2 manipulation in C57BL/6 mice. Upon stimulation with Ag, however, a minor fraction of anti-NP antibodies produced by C57BL6 mice expressed NPa specificities [Boersch-Supan et al., 1985]. These antibodies may use the germline gene V130 [Bothwell, 1984] which was found in anti-NP antibodies of low affinity by Maizels and Bothwell [1985]. This clearly indicates therefore that this gene may be functional as a BALB/c equivalent in C57BL/6. We injected BALB/c Ab2 anti-idiotypic antibodies of the GAT cascade into C57BL/6 mice to check whether the BALB/c H10 equivalent (V130) would then contribute to B6-Ab3 antibodies [Corbet et al., 1988]. It turned out that allogeneic stimulation led to the production of Ab3/Ab1′ antibodies that used the same specific B6 repertoire as did the Ab1. This was true both for the VH and the Vκ chains (fig. 5, 6). This observation therefore suggested that the VH-Vκ pairs were both selected by the GAT antigen or the Ab2 anti-idiotypic antibodies were the same and were strictly strain dependent. As the BALB/c equivalent of H10 is present in C57BL/6, this cannot be attributed simply to a 'hole' in the repertoire. Some other selective pressure must have favored the expression of this pair as opposed to the discrete one which is used by BALB/c mice.

Structural Basis for the pGAT Specificities

The above observations strengthened the degeneracy of sequences that participate in the constitution of the idiotopes in the GAT system, which appear as essentially dependent upon some strain-specific association of discrete VH-Vκ pairs. An approach to the structural correlates, however, remains possible if one restricts oneself to the detailed analysis of a well-defined system, which can be described within a given mouse strain. This was attempted in the BALB/c strain, involving two approaches, one using immunization with synthetic peptides, the other based on common utilization of the 'GAT-specific' VH and Vκ genes by anti-alprenolol antibodies, which did or did not cross-react with the GAT idiotypic mosaic.

Approach of the Structural Correlates of the pGAT Idiotopes by Immunization with Synthetic Peptides

This approach was initiated on the grounds of observed disjunction between idiotype-anti-idiotype interactions and antigen recognition, as already mentioned above for the GAT system. The essence of the disjunction relies on two convergent observations:

(i) Most Ab3 antibodies of the GAT cascade express similar pGAT idiotopes to Ab1. However, only a fraction of these Ab3-Id$^+$ antibodies were, in addition, able to recognize the GAT original antigen, being thus of the Ab1′ type, defined as Id$^+$Ig$^+$. The only structural difference between Ab3-Id$^+$Ag$^-$ and Ab3/Ab1′-Id$^+$Ag$^+$ was found within the D region, the Ab1′ antibodies expressing D regions that had the main structural features defined in Ab1 antibodies, i.e. the presence of aromatic residues most often associated with basic amino acid residues, providing a positive net charge. The organization of the D region so defined was fully consistent with the structure

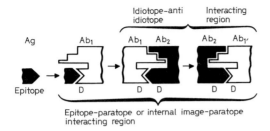

Fig. 7. The clutch model for Ag/Ab1/Ab2/Ab1' interactions, stressing the disjunction between the D region and the other hypervariable regions.

of the dominant epitope of the GAT antigen, mostly centered on Glu and Tyr residues. Residues contributing to the pGAT specificities should therefore be looked for on the other CDRs of the Ab1/Ab1' molecules, i.e. on stretches of hypervariable regions contained in the VH-Vκ pairs characteristic of the pGAT expression within the BALB/c mouse strain.

(ii) At the Ab2 level, the D region was found to contain an internal image-like structure (either Glu-Glu-Tyr or Tyr-Tyr-Glu) which led to the proposals that D-Ab1-DAb2-DAb1' were 'on line' with antigen recognition, whereas other CDRs – at least some of them – were rather involved in idiotype-anti-idiotype interactions. This was most simply expressed as the 'clutch' model of Ig-Ig interaction [Fougereau et al., 1988], represented in figure 7.

Immunization with Ab2-D Synthetic Peptides

Peptides reproducing one of either characteristic Ab2-D region sequences were synthesized and coupled to KLH [Mazza et al., 1985]. Immunization of BALB/c mice led to the occurrence of antibodies that recognized the immunizing peptides. A fraction of these polyclonal antibodies was shown to bind the GAT antigen. These antibodies did not express the pGAT specificities, and were thus classified as Id⁻Ag⁺, bringing further evidence of the disjunction between idiotype and antigen recognition. One monoclonal antibody was isolated, and was also of the Id⁻Ag⁺ type. Sequencing of the mRNA κ-chain indicated that this mAb used a Vκ gene completely different from K5.1 or K1A5 which condition expression of the pGAT idiotype.

Synthetic Peptides Derived from the Ab1 CDR Sequences May Elicit Anti-Ab1 Antibodies. Peptides corresponding to the sequence of the six CDRs of the germline basic anti-GAT mAb1 were synthesized, coupled to KLH, and injected into BALB/c mice [Mazza et al., 1987]. With the exception of CDR1 of the light chains, all peptides stimulated the production of antibodies that were shown to be devoid of any cross-reactivity between the different CDRs. Recognition by these antibodies of the corresponding native CDR determinants on the anti-GAT mAb1 reference molecule was looked for, using direct binding to mAb1-Fab coupled to Sepharose. It was observed that all antisera which had an activity towards the immunizing antigen were also able to bind the native molecule, bringing direct evidence that the mosaic of the pGAT idiotopes could indeed be assigned to the various hypervariable regions of the VH-Vκ pair defining the Ab1 idiotype.

Idiotypic Cross-Reactivity of Anti-GAT and Anti-Alprenolol Antibodies. Recently, Nahmias et al. [1988] reported that some anti-alprenolol (or 'anti-Alp') antibodies used one or the other, or both the VH and Vκ genes used in the GAT system. Three anti-Alp antibodies were of particular interest for contributing to the elucidation of the structural correlates of the pGAT idiotypic mosaic. Two, termed 14C3 and 17C1, used both the VH and the Vκ genes defining the 'GAT' system but did not express any of the pGAT idiotopes. Comparison of the V-D-J regions is given in figure 8. It can first be observed that CDR3 differed extensively between anti-GAT and anti-Alp antibodies, with a drastic change in net charge, reinforcing the importance of the D region in antigen recognition and making it unlikely that it may directly contribute to the respective idiotopes. The sequences encoded by the VH H10 gene were quite conserved, except for 4 positions of substitution that were clustered in CDR2. This observation therefore points to a critical contribution of this hypervariable region to the pGAT idiotopes, in agreement with the observations made in other idiotypic systems, and particularly for the DEX J558 correlates [Clevinger et al., 1980).

Regarding the light chain sequences (fig. 9), anti-Alp are clearly very close from the 'GAT' K5.1 germline gene, which directly encodes Ab1 (51.5.2) and Ab1' (22.186) of the GAT cascade. One to three differences were seen in anti-Alp antibodies within CDR1, where substitutions were also present in some anti-GAT Ab1 (fig. 9), suggesting that this region may tolerate some substitutions without affecting expression of the pGAT idiotopes. CDR1, therefore, may not contribute to idiotypy in the GAT system. In CDR2, a clear-cut difference between anti-GAT and anti-Alp may be seen at position 50, for which the drastic replacement of one basic by an acidic amino acid might greatly influence the three-dimensional structure of this

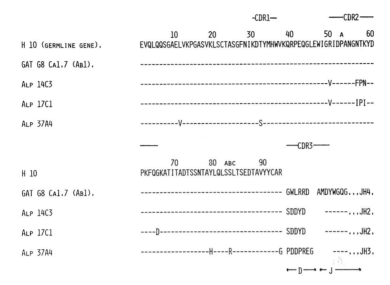

```
                                            -CDR1-           ——CDR2——
                           10        20        30        40      50  A    60
H 10 (GERMLINE GENE).    EVQLQQSGAELVKPGASVKLSCTASGFNIKDTYMHWVKQRPEQGLEWIGRIDPANGNTKYD

GAT G8 CA1.7 (AB1).      ------------------------------------------------------------

ALP 14C3                 -----------------------------------------------V------FPN--

ALP 17C1                 -----------------------------------------------V------IPI--

ALP 37A4                 ----------V--------------------S-----------------------------


                           ——                          ——CDR3——
                           70        80   ABC    90
H 10                     PKFQGKATITADTSSNTAYLQLSSLTSEDTAVYYCAR

GAT G8 CA1.7 (AB1).      ------------------------------------ GWLRRD  AMDYWGQG...JH4.

ALP 14C3                 ------------------------------------ SDDYD      ------...JH2.

ALP 17C1                 ----D------------------------------- SDDYD      ------...JH2.

ALP 37A4                 ------------------H----R------------G PDDPREG    ----...JH3.
                                                              ←—D—→ ←—J—→
```

Fig. 8. Heavy chain variable region amino acid sequence of anti-GAT and anti-alprenolol antibodies using the H10 germline gene.

```
                                           ——CDR1——            ─CDR2─
                           10        20    ABCDE 30       40        50        60
VK5.1 (GERMLINE GENE).   DVVMTQTPLSLPVSLGDQASISCRSSQSLVHSNGNTYLHWYLQKPGQSPKLLIYKVSNRFSGVPD

GAT H51.5.2 (AB1)        ----------------------------------------------------------------
GAT 22.186 (AB1')        ----------------------------------------------------------------
GAT G8 CA1.7 (AB1)       -------------------------I---------Y---------------R----------

ALP 14C3                 ---L-------------------------K-----H------------E----------
ALP 17C1                 ---L-------------------------I-----H------------E----------


                                           ——CDR3——
                           70        80        90
VK5.1.                   RFSGSGSGTDFTLKISRVEAEDLGVYFCSQSTHVP

GAT H51.5.2.             ------------------------------K-I-
GAT 22.186.              ----------------------------------- HTFGGGTKLEIKR  ( JK2 ).
GAT G8 CA1.7             ----------------------M---Y-F-G---- ------------   ( JK2 ).

ALP 14C3                 -------------------------------PW------------ ( JK1 ).
ALP 17C1                 -------------------------------PW------------ ( JK1 ).
```

Fig. 9. Light chain variable region amino acid sequence of anti-GAT and anti-alprenolol antibodies utilizing the VK5.1 germline gene.

region, but is possibly associated with antigen recognition, for the reason already discussed for the D region. Finally, looking at the structure of the third CDR of the light chain points to the presence of an additional proline residue, expressed in the two anti-Alp antibodies (14C3 and 17C1), as the result of a differential junctional diversity using a Vκ-Jκ1 rearrangement, in contrast to the Vκ-Jκ2 combination encountered in anti-GAT antibodies. This region appears therefore as a serious candidate to contribute to the pGAT idiotopes.

Conversely, a third anti-Alp antibody, 22C4. contains a light chain which uses the VK5.1-Jκ2 genes, as do the anti-GAT antibodies. This anti-Alp Ab was found to express only part of the pGAT epitopes, which is best explained by the fact that its heavy chain was encoded by a gene of the 36-60 family [Nahmias et al., 1989], very different from H10, a member of the J558 family, The common epitopes must therefore be contributed to by the light chain which is likely to express a CDR3 very close to that of anti-GAT antibodies because of the VK5.1-JK2 rearrangement.

Taken together, these different comparisons allow us to propose that H-CDR2 and L-CDR3 must contribute to the constitution of the pGAT idiotypic determinants.

General Conclusions

Extensive analysis of the GAT idiotypic cascade has shown several key points in delineating the genetic and structural basis for the idiotypic network. The pGAT public idiotypic determinants are expressed as the result of the combination of a VH-Vκ pair that has been identified at the germline level in the BALB/c mouse. Most Ab1 and Ab3 (Id$^+$Ag$^-$ and Id$^+$Ag$^+$ or Ab1') have sequences which are directly germline encoded by one VH gene, H10, and two very closely related Vκ genes, K5.1 and K1A5. The D region, which appears strongly conserved, and presumably results from a direct germline expression in some cases, plays a major role in antigen recognition, but does not seem to contribute to the idiotypic specificities.

The existence of conserved V-D-J and Vκ-Jκ structures at the Ab2 level also reinforces the germline (or very close to it) nature of this idiotypic cascade, an observation that may be the indication that such networks may play an important role in the selection of the initial repertoire [Fougereau and Schiff, 1988].

Comparison of anti-Alp and anti-GAT antibodies also provided convincing evidence that CDR2 of the heavy chains and CDR3 of the light chains played a key role in the pGAT idiotype expression. One should, however, bear in mind, in view of the analysis of the pGAT expression by the C57BL/6 strain which uses very different VH andf Vκ genes, that the approach of the structural correlates of idiotypy must be confined within a well-defined system, since extensive differences in amino acid sequence may lead to the occurrence of similarly three-dimensionally organized structures that are recognized by the same anti-idiotypic reagent. This is an additional example of the fact that the huge diversity of antibodies cannot escape a compromise between specificity and degeneracy.

Acknowledgments

This work was supported by INSERM (Institut National de la Santé et de la Recherche médicale), and CNRS (Centre national de la recherche scientifique).

References

Boersch-Supan, M.E.; Agarwal, S.; White-Scharf, M.E.; Imanishi-Kari, T.: Heavy chain variable region multiple gene segments encode anti-4 (hydroxy-3-nitrophenyl) acetyl idiotypic antibodies. J. exp. Med. 161: 1272–1292 (1985).

Bothwell, A.L.M.: The genes encoding anti-NP antibodies in inbred strains of mice; in Greene, Nisonoff, The biology of idiotypes, pp. 19–34 (Plenum Press, New York 1984).

Bothwell, A.L.M.; Paskind, M.; Reth, M.; Imanishi-Kari, T.; Rajewsky, K.; Baltimore, D.: Heavy chain variable region contribution to the NP^b family of antibodies. Somatic mutations evident in a γ2a variable region. Cell 24: 625–637 (1981).

Cazenave. P.A.: Idiotypic-anti-idiotypic regulation of antibody synthesis in rabbits. Proc. natn. Acad. Sci. USA 74: 5122–5125 (1977).

Clevinger, B.; Schilling, J.; Hood, L.; Davie, J.M.: Structural correlates of cross-reactive and individual idiotypic determinants on murine antibodies to α(1-3) dextran. J. exp. Med. 151: 1059–1070 (1980).

Corbet, S.; Hirn, M.; Roth, C.; Thèze, J.; Fougereau, M.; Schiff, C.: Allogeneic manipulation of the GAT idiotypic cascade. Immunization of C57BL/6 mice by BALB/c anti-idiotypes stimulates similar strain-specific Vκ genes as the original antigen. J. Immun. 141: 779–784 (1988),

Corbet, S.; Milili, M.; Fougereau, M.; Schiff, C.: Two V germline genes related to the GAT idiotypic network (Ab1 and Ab3/Ab1′) account for the major subfamilies of the mouse Vκ-1 variability subgroup. J. Immun. 138: 932–939 (1987).

Fougereau, M.; Cambillau, C.; Corbet, S.; Mazza, G.; Milili, M.; Moinier, D.; Ollier, P.; Rocca-Serra, J.; Roth, C.; Schiff, C.; Sommé, G.; Thèze, J.; Tonnelle, C.: Molecular basis of anti-Id antibodies carrying internal image of antigens; in Bona, Biological applications of anti-idiotypes, pp. 23–40 (CRC Press, Boca Raton 1988).

Fougereau, M.; Schiff, C.: Breaking the first circle. Immunol. Rev. *105:* 69–84 (1988).

Jerne, N.K.: Towards a network theory of the immune system. Ann. Immunol., Paris *125C:* 373–389 (1974).

Jerne, N.K.; Roland, J.; Cazenave, P.A.: Recurrent idiotopes and internal images. Eur. molec. Biol. Org. J. *1:* 243–247 (1982).

Ju, S.T.; Pierres, M.; Waltenbaugh, C.; Germain, R.N.; Benacerraf, B.; Dorf, M.E.: Idiotypic analysis of monoclonal antibodies to poly ($Glu^{60}Ala^{30}Tyr^{10}$). Proc. natn. Acad. Sci. USA *76:* 2942–2946 (1979).

Loh, D.Y.; Bothwell, A.L.M.; White-Scharf, M.E.; Imanishi-Kari, T.; Baltimore, D.: Molecular basis of a mouse strain-specific anti-hapten response. Cell *33:* 85–93 (1983).

Maizels, N.; Bothwell, A.L.M.: The T-cell independent immune response to the hapten NP uses a large repertoire of heavy chain genes. Cell *43:* 715 (1985).

Mazza, G.; Guigou, V.; Moinier, D.; Corbet, S.; Ollier, P.; Fougereau, M.: Molecular interactions in the 'GAT' idiotypic network. An approach using synthetic peptides. Annls Inst. Pasteur/Immunol., Paris *138:* 3–17 (1987).

Mazza, G.; Ollier, P.; Sommé, G.; Moinier, D.; Rocca-Serra, J.; Van Rietschoten, J.; Thèze, J.; Fougereau, M.: A structural basis for the internal image in the idiotypic network. Antibodies against synthetic Ab2-D regions cross-react with the original antigen. Annls Inst. Pasteur/Immunol., Paris *136D:* 259–269 (1985).

Nahmias, C.; Cazaubon, S.; Strosberg, A.D.: A rabbit antiserum detects a VH J558 subgroup marker highly expressed among anti-alprenolol antibodies. J. Immun. (in press, 1989).

Nahmias, C.; Strosberg, A.D.; Emorine, L.J.: The immune response towards β-adrenergic ligands and their receptors. VIII. Extensive diversity of VH and VL genes encoding anti-alprenolol antibodies. J. Immun. *140:* 1304–1311 (1988).

Ollier, P.; Rocca-Serra, J.; Sommé, G.; Thèze, J.; Fougereau, M.: The idiotypic network and the internal image. Possible regulation of a germ-line network by paucigene-encoded Ab2 (antiidiotypic) antibodies in the GAT system. Eur. molec. Biol. Org. J. *4:* 3681–3688 (1985).

Rocca-Serra, J.; Matthes, H.W.; Kaartinen, M.; Milstein, C.; Thèze, J.; Fougereau, M.: Analysis of antibody diversity. V-D-J mRNA nucleotide sequence of four anti-GAT monoclonal antibodies. A paucigene system using alternate D-J recombinations to generate functionally similar hypervariable regions. Eur. molec. Biol. Org. J.. *2:* 867–872 (1983a).

Rocca-Serra, J.; Tonnelle, C.; Fougereau, M.: Two monoclonal antibodies against different antigens use the same VH germ-line gene. Nature, Lond. *304:* 353–355 (1983b).

Roth, C.; Rocca-Serra, J.; Sommé, G.; Fougereau, M.; Thèze, J.: Gene repertoire of the anti-poly ($Glu^{60}Ala^{30}Tyr^{10}$) (GAT) immune response. Comparison of VH, Vκ and D regions used by anti-GAT antibodies and monoclonal antibodies produced after antiidiotypic immunization. Proc. natn. Acad. Sci. USA *182:* 4788–4797 (1985a).

Roth, C.; Sommé, G.; Schiff, C.; Thèze, J.: Immune response against GAT. Immunization with monoclonal antiidiotypic antibodies leads to the predominant stimulation of idiotypically similar Ig with an anti-GAT activity. Eur. J. Immunol. *15:* 576–580 (1985b).

Schiff, C.; Milili, M.; Fougereau, M.: Immunoglobulin diversity. Analysis of the germ-line VH gene repertoire of the murine anti-GAT response. Nucl. Acids Res. *11:* 4007–4017 (1983).

Schiff, C.; Milili, M.; Hue, I.; Rudikoff, S.; Fougereau, M.: Genetic basis for expression of the idiotypic network. One unique Ig VH germline gene accounts for the major family of Ab1 and Ab3 (Ab1′) antibodies of the GAT system. J. exp. Med. *163:* 573–587 (1986).

Schnurr, I.: Idiotypes, antigens on the inside. Workshop at the Basel Institute for Immunology, p. 122 (Hoffman-La Roche, Basel 1981).

Sommé, G.; Roth, C.; Mazie, J.C.; Salem, P.; Thèze, J.: Public and individual idiotopes in the anti-GAT response. Analysis by monoclonal antibodies. Eur. J. Immunol. *13:* 1023–1030 (1983).

Takemori, T.; Tesch, H.; Reth, M.; Rajewsky, K.: The immune response against anti-idiotype antibodies. I. Induction of idiotype bearing antibodies and analysis of the idiotope repertoire. Eur. J. Immunol. *12:* 1040–1010 (1982).

Thèze, J.; Moreau, J.L.: Genetic control of the immune response to the GAT terpolymer. I. Interstrain and interspecies cross-reactive idiotype. Ann. Immunol., Paris *129C:* 721–726 (1978).

Urbain, J.; Wikler, M.; Franssen, J.D.; Collignon, C.: Idiotypic regulation of the immune system by the induction of antibodies against anti-idiotypic antibodies. Proc. natn. Acad. Sci. USA *74:* 5126–5130 (1977).

Michel Fougereau, DVM, Dr Sc, Centre d'Immunologie INSERM-CNRS de Marseille-Luminy, Case 906, F-13288 Marseille Cedex 9 (France)

Carson DA, Chen PP, Kipps TJ (eds): Idiotypes in Biology and Medicine.
Chem Immunol. Basel, Karger, 1990, vol 48, pp 30–48

Structural Implications of AB2s

Are Novel D Segments Involved with Anti-Idiotypic Specificity?

Katheryn Meek, J. Donald Capra

Department of Microbiology, University of Texas Southwestern Medical School,
Dallas, Tex., USA

Introduction

In 1974, Jerne [1] proposed that the immune response might be regulated via the unique antigenic determinants of immunoglobulin variable regions (idiotypes) described earlier by Kunkel et al. [2] and Oudin and Michel [3]. This hypothesis predicts that the idiotypic determinants of each antibody molecule would be complemented by those of another, creating an idiotypic network through which immunoglobulin expression might be controlled. A multitude of experiments has followed in which manipulation of the immune response was achieved through the use of anti-idiotypic reagents [4]. These studies have generally strengthened his hypothesis.

Jerne extended his ideas in 1982 by grouping Ab2s into two functional subsets: those that recognize determinants present in the V region and which do not involve the combining site for the eliciting antigen, and those that represent internal images of the eliciting antigen [5]. He also proposed that naturally occurring Ab2s exist which represent internal images of exogenous antigens, and that these antibodies are important in the establishment of the B cell repertoire. Thus, the idiotypic network might not only be functionally important in the regulation of immune responses, but may also play a role in the establishment of the preimmune repertoire.

Anti-idiotypic antibodies of both types have been described by several groups in many systems [6, 7]. However, since the antibody repertoire appears to be complete in its capacity to respond to protein antigens, the mere existence of anti-idiotypic antibodies does not necessarily infer their relevance. Certainly, immunoglobulin molecules are excellent examples of protein immunogens. Thus, the physiologic significance of the idiotypic network continues to be a source of debate.

Jerne's network theory can most simply be illustrated as follows:

Antigen--> Ab1 <--> Ab2 <--> Ab3 <--> ...etc.

He suggested that complementary sets of V regions might be generated directly from the germline, independent of somatic variation. Indeed, it seems logical that if the interaction between Abls and Ab2s is crucial to the function of the immune system, then their generation should not be random. It follows that if in a particular antigenic system, the majority of Abls elicited are structurally homogeneous, then the Ab2s within that system should be similar structurally as well.

Hapten systems are ideal for approaching the question of a germline-encoded network for several reasons. Unlike the responses to more complex protein antigens, the primary responses to haptens are more homogeneous. In addition, since hapten systems have been used extensively in studying all aspects of immunoglobulin structure and function, the Ab1 responses in these systems are the best characterized to date. Finally, Abls elicited in response to many of the haptenic antigens are encoded directly in the germline and bear strong cross-reactive idiotypes. It is not coincidental then, that most of our knowledge of structural characteristics of anti-idiotypic antibodies (the focus of this chapter) comes from the hapten systems.

At this time we are limited to the published information generated in the following systems: NP, GAT, Ars, PC, and reovirus [8–13]. There is also partial structural information on Ab2s in the 3-fucosyl lactosamine, and dextran systems [14]. A total of 32 Ab2 structures (some syngeneic and some allogeneic) have been reported. In one case, three of the antibodies may have been clonal duplicates; two antibodies in another case may have been clonally related. Thus, 29 distinct Ab2 structures have been completed.

Studies in the Anti-NP System

Sablitzky and Rajewsky [8] were the first to report detailed structural information on a group of anti-idiotypic antibodies. The response of the C57BL/6 strain to the hapten (4-hydroxy-3-nitro-phenyl)acetyl (NP) is a homogeneous response consisting primarily of antibodies derived from a single heavy chain variable region gene segment and a single lambda variable region gene segment [15, 16]. The heavy and light chain variable regions of six syngeneic monoclonal Ab2s in this system have been completely sequenced. The antibodies were derived in two ways: four from fusions of spleen cells from mice immunized with a monoclonal anti-NP antibody representing the unmutated C57BL/6 germline anti-NP antibody, and two from mice immunized with an antibody derived from the same C57BL/6 anti-NP gene with several somatic mutations.

The two Ab2s derived by immunizing with the somatic variant use identical germline gene segments (V_H, D, J_H, V_K, J_K) and may be clonally related. This V_H segment is homologous to the V_H segment of one of the Ab2s derived by immunizing with the germline Ab1, but the rest of the variable regions (D, J_H, V_K, and J_K) in this Ab2 are distinct from those in any of the other five Ab2s. Two of the four antibodies recognizing germline anti-NP molecules apparently derive from the same V_K, V_H, and D gene segments. One NP Ab2 uses germline gene segments entirely distinct from those employed by any of the other Ab2s.

The following conclusions can be drawn from this work: First, somatic mutation is apparent in anti-idiotypic antibodies. This can be concluded (even though the C57BL/6 germline genes from which these molecules derive have not been identified) because there are sequence variations between very closely related Ab2s which presumably derive from the same germline elements. In addition, sequence variations are apparent in the joining and diversity segments of these molecules when compared to the Balb/c published germline sequences. (It is possible that the C57BL/6 differs in J_H, D and J_K from Balb/c.) Second, the third complementarity-determining regions of these antibodies are not derived from the germline. Three of the heavy chains have third CDRs which are unusually long (15 amino acid residues). Only a portion of these are derived from known germline D elements. One of these Ab2s derives its D segments from a known germline D element, but it is translated in an altered reading frame from that usually seen in heavy chain diversity segments. In contrast to T cell receptor D segments, immunoglobulin D segments have a favored reading frame. However, in some instances (perhaps as often as 10%) the D segment in an expressed antibody is translated in one of the other two (not preferred) reading frames [17]. The other three antibodies have D segments of a more typical length, but these are also not generated directly from known germline elements. Finally, syngeneic Ab2s in the NP system are closely related structurally to each other and appear to derive from a limited number of germline gene segments.

Serologically, in the NP system, the isogenic anti-idiotypic response is weak [18, 19]. Weak serologic Ab2 responses have been reported in several other systems as well. One possible explanation is that unusual D segments may be required for Ab2 specificity. The generation of unusual D segments may require multiple somatic processes, and, therefore, may be infrequently generated. So, antibodies with this particular specificity would rarely be found in the repertoire. Information implying that the potential anti-idiotypic repertoire is actually quite large would not support this conclusion [20, 21]. Alternatively, weak expression of syngeneic anti-idiotypic responses could be due to some type of active suppression.

Studies in the Anti-GAT System

The most extensive description of anti-idiotypic antibodies within a single system was published in 1985 by Ollier et al. [9]. They described a panel of syngeneic monoclonal anti-idiotypic antibodies which were derived from mice immunized with either monoclonal or polyclonal Balb/c anti-GAT antibodies expressing the public cGAT idiotype [9]. When monoclonal Ab1s served as the immunogen, Ab2s were isolated which recognized private idiotopes only. When polyclonal anti-GAT antibodies were used as the immunogen, the Ab2s isolated recognized public GAT idiotopes. The Ab2s which recognized public idiotopes fell into two groups serologically. One group recognizes public idiotopes of the anti-GAT response in several strains of mice. The second group recognizes public idiotopes present nearly exclusively on Balb/c anti-GAT antibodies.

Structurally, the anti-idiotypic antibodies recognizing private GAT idiotopes are distinct, all deriving from completely different variable region gene segments. This is in direct contrast to what is observed in the antibodies recognizing public GAT idiotopes. Within each of the two serologic groups (although isolated from separate fusions) the antibodies are nearly identical to each other, deriving from the same V_H, D, J_H, V_K, and J_K gene segments. It is clear that somatic mutation occurs in GAT Ab2s.

The third complementarity-determining regions of the heavy chains of these molecules are very interesting for several reasons. They are extremely long – 16 or 17 amino acids. None can be explained completely from any of the published germline D sequences. The D segments in two of the Ab2s appear to have resulted from a double inverted fusion of two DSP2 D segments (fig. 1). The 5' portion of this D segment appears to have derived

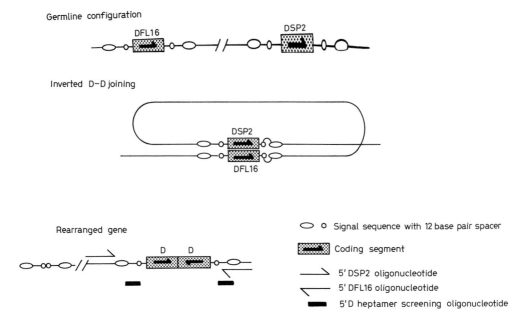

Germline configuration

DFL16 DSP2

Inverted D–D joining

DSP2

DFL16

Rearranged gene

D D

○ ○ Signal sequence with 12 base pair spacer

▓▓▓ Coding segment

⟶ 5′ DSP2 oligonucleotide

⟍ 5′ DFL16 oligonucleotide

▬ 5′D heptamer screening oligonucleotide

Fig. 1. Diagrammatic model of inverted D to D joining. Coding regions and recombination signal sequences are as indicated.

			L	I	P	F	S	D	G	Y	Y	E	D
HP22			TTA	ATC	CCT	TTC	TCT	GAT	GGT	TAC	TAC	GAG	GAC
HP27			---	---	---	---	---	---	---	---	---	---	---
DSP2.(2,3,4)						--	-AC	T--	---	---	---	G--	
cDSP2.(2,3,4)	TAG	-AG	---	---	-								

Fig. 2. Nucleotide and deduced amino acid sequences of the D region of monoclonal GAT anti-idiotypic antibodies. A line indicates homology to the reference sequences of known germline D sequences. The reverse complement of a particular sequence is indicated by a 'c' before the name.

from the noncoding strand of one DSP2 D segment, the next seventeen base pairs are identical to the coding strand of another of the DSP2 D segments. Ollier et al. [9] proposed an inverted recombination between the coding strand of one of the DSP2 D segments (using the alternative signal sequences proposed by Kurosawa and Tonegawa [22]) and the noncoding strand of a second DSP2 D segment (fig. 2). A second inverted recombination would then occur between J_H and the 5' portion of the noncoding strand, reinstating the normal orientation between D and J_H. Finally, V_H to D rearrangement would occur between the 3' portion of V_H and the now fused D segments. A similar mechanism has been hypothesized to account for the conserved N segment seen in many murine anti-arsonate antibodies [23]. Recently inverted and direct D-D fusion intermediates (before rearrangement to J_H or V_H) have been isolated from bone marrow DNA demonstrating that this mechanism actually occurs [24]. It is quite striking that the same unusual D segment occurs in two independently derived anti-idiotypic antibodies. The most straightforward explanation is that this particular D segment is selected for by antigen (Ab1s), implying that this structure is important for function.

Perhaps the most interesting aspect of the D segments of these molecules is the presence of sequences which appear to mimic the structure of the original antigen – the random terpolymer GAT (glu-ala-tyr). The proposed internal image occurs in the D segments of both groups of public anti-idiotopes as well as in the D segment of one private anti-idiotope. The sequence glu-glu-tyr is present in the D regions of two Ab2s; whereas the sequence tyr-tyr-glu is present in the D regions of three other Ab2s. It has been shown that the glu-tyr residues of the GAT terpolymer are the most important for antigen binding of GAT Ab1s.

Studies in the Anti-Arsonate System

In the Ars system, our laboratory has structurally characterized seven monoclonal anti-idiotypic antibodies recognizing distinct public idiotopes which in part comprise the cross-reactive idiotype (CRI_A) associated with the A/J strain's response to the hapten, para-azophenylarsonate [11, 12, 14]. In contrast to the previous two studies, 4 of the 7 Ars Ab2s described are allogeneic. These Ab2s were isolated from Balb/c mice (a strain which normally does not express the CRI_A) immunized with polyclonal, idiotype-positive, A/J anti-arsonate antibodies, and then boosted with a monoclonal anti-arsonate antibody [25]. The other three Ab2s studied are syngeneic, isolated from A/J mice immunized with polyclonal A/J idiotype positive anti-arsonate antibodies [26].

The allogeneic Ab2 response is structurally heterogeneous – deriving from several different gene segments. This heterogeneity is also apparent serologically – each Ab2 recognizes a different idiotypic determinant. The amino acid residues in the A/J Ab1s affecting expression of each of these four idiotopes has been determined through sequence information, chemical modifications, and chain recombination experiments [27]. The expression of three of the idiotopes is most dependent on amino acid residues located in the D region of the Ab1s, whereas the expression of one idiotope is heavily influenced by the amino acid in position 59 of the heavy chain variable region. These allogeneic Ab2s are actually representative of what one would expect in an antibody response to any foreign protein – deriving from many different germline elements directed against many different antigenic determinants present on the immunogen.

The most striking feature of this study is the extreme heterogeneity of allogeneic Ab2s compared to the near identity of the syngeneic Ab2s [14]. Four allogeneic Ab2s derive from different V_H, D, J_H, V_K and J_K gene segments. In contrast, the three syngeneic Ab2s are nearly identical to one another. Clonal relatedness of the three cannot formally be ruled out. Certainly (as is the case in NP and GAT), the syngeneic Ab2 response in the Ars system is serologically weak, and is limited in its use of germline gene segments.

It is interesting to note the high number of hydrophilic residues – especially negatively charged residues (as is the original antigen, Ars) in the D segments of the allogeneic Ab2s. Of particular interest is the D segment of the Ab2, 2D3. This Ab2 defines an idiotope which is strongly affected by position 59 in the heavy chains of the Ab1s. All Ab1s which have a lysine in this position express this idiotope, whereas Ab1s with any other amino acid in position 59 lack expression of this idiotope. The D segments of this Ab2 begins with three aspartic acid residues (fig. 3). Since at physiologic pH lysine is positively charged, and aspartic acid is negatively charged, it is possible that some of the idiotope-anti-idiotope interactions may be ionic in nature.

The D segments of the three syngeneic molecules are average in length in contrast to the unusual length of the D segments of GAT and NP Ab2s. However, as was the case in the GAT Ab2s, they were probably generated by inverted D-D fusion (fig. 3). Each is 14 base pairs long. The first six appear to be derived from the noncoding strand of DFL16.1; the next six appear to be from the coding strand of DSP2.6. We propose a similar mechanism as suggested by Ollier et al. [9] in the GAT system to generate this unusual sequence. We hypothesize that an inverted recombination event occurs between the coding strand of one D segment and the noncoding strand of the second [14]. Since the syngeneic molecules in this study may be clonally related, it is impossible to determine whether or not the event generating this

```
                              G    S    G    S    S
E4                            GGA  TCC  GGT  AGT  AGC
DFL16.1                    AT TAC  -C-  ---  ---  ---


                              D    S    H    C    G    Q    A
E3                            GAT  AGC  CAC  TGT  GGC  CAG  GC
DSP2.3                             TC   T--  -A-  --T  T-C  -AC


                              D    D    D    G    S
2D3                           GAT  GAT  GAT  GGT  TCC
DSP2.4                             TC   T-C  T--  ---  -A-  GAC
DSP2.2                     TC TAC  T--  ---  T-C  -AC


                              G    X    I    M    Y    G    S    Y
H8                            GGG  XAT  ATA  ATG  TAT  GGT  AGC  TAT
cDFL16.2                   GTA -CC  GTA  G--  ---  A-
DSP2.7                                    CC   TAC  ---  ---  -A-  --C


                              N    E    G    Y    A
12S18-1                       AAT  GAA  GGT  TAC  GCC
12S28-16                      ---  ---  ---  ---  ---
12S84-3                       ---  ---  ---  ---  ---
cDFL16.2            GT  AGC  CGT  AGT  ---  ---
DSP2.6                             CC   TAC  T-T  ---  ---  -A-
```

Fig. 3. Nucleotide and deduced amino acid sequences of the D region of monoclonal arsonate anti-idiotypic antibodies. A line indicates homology to the reference sequences of known germline D sequences. The reverse complement of a particular sequence is indicated by a 'c' before the name.

unusual D segment occurs repeatedly in Ab2s in the arsonate system, as is the case in the GAT system.

The D segment of the four allogeneic Ab2s are also not easily explained from existing germline gene segments. D-D fusion may be invoked to explain 2 of the 4 (fig. 3). It is noteworthy that D-D fusions may best explain the D segments seen in two of the first three Ab2 systems studied.

Since there are no germline sequences available which are more than 95% homologous to the V_H or V_K regions of any of the Ars Ab2s, it is difficult to determine what effect somatic mutation has had on their generation. However, as was the case in both the NP and GAT Ab2s, sequence variation occurs between the variable regions of closely related syngeneic molecules. Limited somatic mutation is apparent in both the J_H and J_K regions of both the syngeneic and allogeneic molecules. Therefore, it seems likely that somatic mutation occurs in both syngeneic and allogeneic arsonate anti-idiotypic antibodies.

Studies in the Anti-Phosphocholine System

Several groups have sequenced allogeneic and syngeneic anti-idio-typic antibodies in the anti-phosphocholine (PC) system [12–14]. The only complete heavy and light chain variable region sequences are those of two allogeneic Ab2s. These antibodies have quite distinct sero-logic reactivites in that the idiotypic specificity of one is hapten inhi-bitable while the other is not [13]. An additional partial heavy chain variable region sequence is available from a third allogeneic Ab2 [12], and three partial heavy chain variable region sequences have been done from syngeneic PC Ab2s [12].

Again, the most striking observation from these studies is the heterogeneity of germline gene use in allogeneic anti-idiotypic anti-bodies as is the case in the allogeneic anti-arsonate Ab2s. The three al-logeneic Ab2s derive their V_H segments from distinct members of the J558 V_H family. The light chain variable regions of two of the three derive from distinct V_K subgroups. The third V_K is not sequenced.

In contrast (with the limited amount of sequence information avail-able), it appears that the syngeneic PC Ab2s are somewhat restricted in their use of germline gene segments. The V_H segments from these Ab2s are nearly identical (at least in their third framework regions). How-ever, unlike the syngeneic Ab2s in the other three systems discussed, the D segments of each syngeneic Ab2 studied in this system is dis-tinct from the others. The light chain variable regions of these syngen-eic Ab2s have not been studied.

Although none of these six Ab2s have D segments wich derive di-rectly from known germline elements, most are easily explained from germline D elements unlike the Ab2 D segments from the other three systems discussed. Two of the allogeneic PC Ab2s have fairly long N segments (13 nucleotides in one; 6 nucleotides in the other) between the V_H and D portions of their heavy chain variable regions. However, each is made up predominantly of guanine nucleotides which terminal transferase presumably prefers [28]. Thus, these N segments can both be explained most easily by nucleotide additions during V_H-D rearran-gement by terminal transferase. As was the case in one of the syngen-eic NP Ab2s, one of the syngeneic PC Ab2s derives its D segments from a known germline D element, but uses it in an altered reading frame. None of the PC Ab2s seem to derive their D segments via D-D fusion.

Studies in the Reovirus System

In 1986, Bruck et al. [10] reported the heavy and light chain variable region sequence of an anti-idiotypic antibody that expresses an internal image of the receptor-binding epitope of the reovirus type 3. The Ab2 was induced syngeneically by immunizing with a monoclonal anti-reovirus Ab1 which expresses a recurrent idiotype. This anti-idiotypic antibody was found to antigenically mimic antigen by several criteria.

The heavy chain variable region of the reovirus Ab2 is nearly identical within the V_H and J_H regions of anti-GAT Ab1s. However, its D segment, as well as its light chain, differ from GAT Ab1s. In addition, the kappa variable region sequence of the reovirus Ab2 is unique from any V_K segment sequenced to date and may represent another V_K family. Since the V_H region is identical (except for one silent substitution) to GAT Ab1s, these findings reinforce Jerne's hypothesis that Ab1 and Ab2 are operational terms in that a single V_H gene segment can generate an Ab1 in one system and Ab2 in another. In this instance, combinatorial diversity explains the two different specificities.

Since the V_H region of this antibody is so similar (only a single silent substitution) to GAT Ab1s, it is likely that they derive from the same germline V_H gene segment which implies that somatic mutation was insignificant in its generation. In addition, the J_H segment is completely germline. The core of the Ab2s D segment (nine nucleotides) derives from a known germline D element, but N segments are apparent at both the V-D and D-J junctions. These most likely derive from terminal transferase nucleotide additions.

The most important observation from this study is that a possible molecular explanation of antigen mimicry by the Ab2 was found. Amino acid sequence comparison between the heavy and light chain variable regions of this Ab2 and reovirus hemagglutinin reveals two significant areas of homology which could account for this phenomenon. There is significant homology between amino acids 317 to 323 of viral hemagglutinin and a nine amino acid sequence at the border of the second framework and the second hypervariable region of the heavy chain variable region. An adjacent region of viral hemagglutinin, amino acids 323 to 332, is significantly homologous to a ten amino acid sequence in the second hypervariable region of the light chain. It is plausible that these two regions in the heavy and light chain variable regions together form an epitope that biologically mimics antigen.

Studies from Other Systems

There are partial heavy chain variable region sequences available from two other systems, anti-3-fucosyl lactosamine (3FL) and antidextran [12]. The most interesting observation from these sequences is from the two syngeneic 3FL Ab2s. As is the case in the PC Ab2s, the V_H regions of these Ab2s apear to be very homologous to one another. However, the D segments and J_H segments are distinct from one another. Again, the D segments of these two Ab2s cannot be easily explained from known germline D elements, but may have been derived by D-D fusion as discussed previously.

There are two partial heavy chain variable region sequences available from the anti-dextran system. Both are syngeneic, and they are structurally different from one another.

Structural Characteristics of Anti-Idiotypic Antibodies

Several important conclusions can be drawn from these studies, if the limitations of the systems are considered. Since the Ab2s studied to date (even within a system) have been generated in a variety of different ways (i.e. by immunizing with polyclonal or monoclonal reagents, etc.), generalizations must be made with caution. Most of the Ab2s which have been studied have come from hapten systems – which may not be representative antigens. It is possible that anti-idiotypic antibodies in other immune responses may differ considerably from the molecules studied thus far. Still, with certain limitations, some important generalities can be drawn. Table 1 summarizes the structural data available to date on anti-idiotypic antibodies.

V Segment Gene Usage Appears to Be Restricted in Syngeneic but Not in Allogeneic Ab2s which Recognize Public Idiotopes

This is best illustrated in the anti-arsonate and anti-PC systems in that syngeneic Ab2s appear to derive from the same or extremely similar germline V_H gene segments, whereas allogeneic Ab2s in both systems are heterogeneous (deriving from dissimilar variable region genes). Furthermore, syngeneic Ab2s recognizing public idiotopes in the anti-NP, anti-GAT, and anti-3FL systems are somewhat restricted in their use of germline V segments. No other allogeneic Ab2s have been studied.

In contrast, syngeneic Ab2s that recognize private idiotopes are not restricted in germline gene usage. This observation is most clearly demon-

Table 1. Summary of available AB2 structures

Name	Syngeneic allotypic	System	V_H family	Length of DH	Length of 5′N	Length of 3′N	Ref. No.
A2597	S	NP	J558	29	3	7	8
A3160	S	NP	J558	29	1	9	8
A3940	S	NP	J558	30	9	8	8
A8/24	S	NP	J558	12	5	2	8
A6/24	S	NP	J558	18	2	3	8
HP22	S	GAT	3660	33	16	6	9
HP27	S	GAT	3660	33	16	6	9
HP20	S	GAT	3660	30	4	20	9
HP21	S	GAT	3660	30	4	9	9
HP25	S	GAT	3660	30	4	9	9
HP9	S	GAT	S107	21	10	0	9
HP12	S	GAT	3660	18	2	6	9
HP13	S	GAT	J558	36	9	6	9
4C11	A	PC	J558	11	0	1	13
F63	A	PC	J558	19	13	0	13
GB4-10	A	PC	J558	18	9	0	14
B3682	S	PC	3609	13	0	4	14
B3938	S	PC	3609	22	4	2	14
B3675	S	PC	–	15	1	3	14
D8-3	S	J558	X24	27	7	5	14
NZO	S	Dex	3660	15	2	1	14
87.92.6	S	Reo	J558	18	4	4	10
E3	A	ARS	3609	20	7	6	14
E4	A	ARS	J558	21	5	0	14
H8	A	ARS	J558	24	12	1	14
2D3	A	ARS	J558	14	7	1	14
12S18–1	S	ARS	J558	14	6	0	14
6C4	S	3FL	7183	18	6	3	14
6B1	S	3FL	7183	26	9	5	14

strated in the GAT system, in which molecules recognizing distinct private idiotopes were completely heterogeneous – while Ab2s recognizing public idiotopes were closely related (more than 95% homologous).

These results in general support Jerne's idea of the coexistence of complementary sets of variable region genes in the germline. Within a single strain, a structurally distinct population appears to induce (or is idiotypic to) a second group of a structurally distinct group of antibodies. The structural dissimilarity of the allogeneic anti-idiotypic antibodies supports this idea. It is not surprising that a strain which lacks a particular variable region gene segment to which an anti-idiotypic response is directed (as is the case in the allogeneic Ars Ab2s), responds as if that antibody were a foreign antigen.

Ab2s Are Not Biased in V_H or V_K Gene Segment Utilization

There is apparently nothing distinct about the V_H or V_K regions of anti-idiotypic antibodies. With the exception of the light chain variable region of the reovirus Ab2, these molecules derive from germline heavy and kappa chain variable genes which can easily be placed within variable region families already described. While the gene segment usage is restricted within a given anti-idiotypic response, the gene usage in general by these antibodies is not biased to any heavy chain variable region or kappa variable region gene family. The strongest evidence for this comes from the reovirus system where the V_H region of the Ab2 is identical (except for one silent substitution) to the V_H region in GAT Ab1s. Thus, it seems certain that Ab2s can be derived from the same pool of V region genes that give rise to Ab1s. This obviously reinforces Jerne's hypothesis that Ab1 and Ab2 are operational terms in that a single V region gene segment can generate an Ab1 in one system and an Ab2 in another.

Six different heavy chain variable region families are represented in this panel of Ab2s. The J558 family is employed most frequently, but this is undoubtedly due to the large size of the J558 family (possibly 1,000 genes) compared to the other V_H gene families (approximately 1–30 genes). There is no apparent bias for proximal (or distal) V_H gene segment usage. Two Ab2s derive from the 7183 V_H gene family (the most 3′) whereas two derive from the 3609 family (the most 5′) [29].

Somatic Variation Occurs in Anti-Idiotypic Antibodies

There are multiple examples of somatic mutation in the joining segments of some (but not all) of these Ab2s. However, since in most cases, the germline genes from which these antibodies derive have not been sequenced, it is impossible to judge to what degree somatic mutation has affected the variable regions of these molecules. In systems where germline V regions are available to compare to expressed sequences, somatic mutation in the J segment parallels that seen in other areas of the variable regions. So it seems probable that somatic mutation plays a role in the generation of at least some Ab2s – as is the case in Ab1s. Even so, since there are many examples of antibodies that have undergone somatic mutation in which specificity is not altered, it remains uncertain whether or not somatic mutation is actually important for any of these antibodies' idiotypic specificities. Indeed, it does not seem surprising that anti-idiotypic antibodies should be affected by the same diversifying mechanisms that affect Ab1s. In any case, it is doubtful that the idiotypic network is strictly germline encoded.

Possible Structural Correlates of Internal Images

One of the most intriguing aspects of studying structures of anti-idiotypic antibodies is attempting to correlate structure with anti-idiotypic specificity. Although definitive evidence of the structural correlate of an antigen mimicking epitope is difficult to obtain, the results of Ollier et al. [9] and Bruck et al [10] are very encouraging. In both of these studies, homologous sequences were demonstrated between antigen and Ab2. These studies involved Ab2s which mimicked antigen, but recent work suggest that noninternal image-bearing Ab2s may be just as effective in perturbing the idiotypic network as those that mimic antigen. Continued study in this area is essential if anti-idiotypic antibodies are to be used to their full potential.

The D Segments of Many Ab2s Are Novel in Structure and Cannot Easily Be Explained by Previously Described Germline D Segments

In more than half the NP^b and GAT Ab2s, the third complementarity-determining regions are extremely long – 15–17 amino acid residues (the third complementarity region in murine heavy chain can vary in length from 7 to 19 amino acids). Although the third CDR in Ab2s from other systems (with a few exceptions) are of a more usual length than those in the GAT and NP^b systems, they do share another structural characteristic – a high percentage of these antibodies appear to have generated their D segments by novel mechanisms. It is striking that in two GAT Ab2s (independently derived), five Ars Ab2s (three possibly clonally related), and two anti-3FL Ab2s, the D segments appear to derive from an unusual inverted D-D fusion. Although a similar mechanism has been proposed to generate the D segments in antibodies that are not anti-idiotypic [23], the proportion of the sequences generated from the inverted fusion was small compared to the proportion generated from germline elements in normal orientation (only one amino acid residue). In contrast, nearly half of the D segments in these Ab2s are derived from the proposed inversion event.

It is possible that as antibodies of more specificites are sequenced, unusual D segments will be seen in Ab1s that have extremely long D segments. There are also examples of D segments in Ab1s that cannot be easily explained by existing germline gene segments and which may have fused D segments [30]. To differentiate whether or not novel D segments are a common structural feature of Ab2s (and therefore possibly relevant to their

Table 2. D segment analysis of antibodies with various specificities

Specificity	Number	Length	% germline	N segments		Ratio GC/AT
				length of 5' N	length of 3' N	
Hapten	34	18.9	67	2.7	2.4	1.7
Unknown	22	17.0	66	2.5	3.4	1.6
Protein	11	12.6	61	2.6	1.4	1.2
Self carbohydrate	4	14.7	60	3.5	2.0	3.4
Self protein	29	14.5	54	3.8	2.6	2.0
Ab2s	29	22.2	52	6.1	4.4	1.2
Ab3s	7	16.2	72	2.1	2.0	2.6

specificity), we have compared D segments from Ab2s to those of Ab1s. First, for each antibody analyzed, the D segment was defined as the portion of the third hypervariable region which could not be accounted for by either the 3' portion of the V_H segment or the 5' portion of the J_H gene utilized. In instances where the germline V_H segment sequence is not available, the 3' portion of V was defined as position 94 (usually arginine) since this is what is observed in heavy chain variable region gene segments. Then, the percentage of each D segment which could be explained by a known germline D segment via simple V_H-D-J_H assembly was determined (i.e. without N segment addition, somatic mutation, or D-D fusion). One hundred Ab1 sequences were included in this analysis [31, 32]. Since in the majority of the antibodies studied at least a portion of the D segment can be explained by one of the previously described germline D elements, we have compared the N segments [12] of these Ab2s to those of Ab1s. We define the N segments as the 3' or 5' portion of the D segment not explained by the germline D segment from which the core of a particular D segment apparently derives. Since N segments are thought to be the result of terminal transferase additions of nucleotides during V_H-D and D-J_H rearrangement, and this enzyme has a preference for C's and G's over A's and T's [28], we have compared not only the length of both the 5' and 3' N segments in these antibodies, but also the relative GC content. If N segment generation in most antibodies is primarily due to terminal transferase, but in other antibodies is the result of some other mechanism, this may be reflected in the relative GC content of their N segments. The results of this comparison are shown in table 2. From this limited analysis, it appears that D segments in anti-idiotypic antibodies are slightly longer than those of Ab1s and this difference in length is primarily due to the 3′ and 5′ N segment additions in these antibodies. This does not directly reflect the length of the third hypervariable region; it simply reflects the percentage of the third hypervariable region derived from the D segment or from N segments additions. Thus, Ab2s derive a larger portion of the third hypervariable region from D and N than do Ab1s. In addition, Ab2s are slightly more homologous to germline D segments than are Ab2s. What is most interesting from this comparison is the difference in relative GC/AT content. In the N segments in most Ab1s this ratio varies from 1.6 to 3.4; whereas in anti-idiotypic antibodies and antiprotein antibodies the ratio of GC/AT is 1.2.

Comparisons like these must be interpreted with caution in that the available immunoglobulin literature is biased towards antibodies with particular specificities. The number of Ab1s in several categories is very low. In addition, it is impossible to correct for the bias (via antigenic selection) the immune system itself places on junctional residues in immunoglobulins. There are several examples of antibodies in which the junctional residues determine the antibody's specificity [33, 34]. The D segments observed in Ab2s may be an example of this selection. However, results like these, in addition to previous reports of conserved N segments [23] and D-D fusion [9, 14, 24] strengthen the idea that mechanisms other than simple terminal transferase additions may play a role in the generation of the third hypervariable region in immunoglobulin heavy chains. Whether or not this is not readily explained through novel mechanisms of rearrangement, still undiscovered D elements within the germline, somatic mutation, or other mechanisms remains to the determined.

There is no obvious reason why novel mechanisms should play more of a role in the generation of antibodies of one specificity than another. It would seem most likely that since D-D fusion does occur in normal animals, it should play a role in the generation of many antibodies. In fact, there are examples of Ab1s in which D-D fusion may have occurred [30]. As antibodies of more specificities are studied, instances of novel D segments or D-D fusion may become more apparent in antibodies of many specificities.

Alternatively, if unusual D segments continue to be observed primarily in anti-idiotypic antibodies it would imply that Ab2s are derived from the germline differently than Ab1s. There is some additional indirect evidence in support of this idea. If the unusual D segments observed in Ab2s were in any way artifactual, it would seem logical that the same artifact should be seen in generating Ab3s. There have been a very limited number of Ab3s sequenced [35]; novel D segments have not been observed (table 2) strengthening the observation that novel D segments may be peculiar to Ab2s. This may force a considerable alteration in our present thinking of idiotypic networks.

It is tempting to speculate on the possible importance of novel D segments to anti-idiotypic antibodies. The majority of syngeneic anti-idiotypic responses are very weak. If novel D segments are necessary for the Ab2s specificities, and the event that generates these structures represents a relatively rare rearrangement, then antibodies with the appropriate specificity would be rare in the B cell repertoire and their expression would be only at a low level. However, this unusual rearrangement mechanism may actually be common. In fact, before any Ab2s were sequenced, several investigators made the observation that though isogenic anti-idiotypic responses are weak, the potential repertoire of B cells expressing anti-idiotypic determinants is relatively large [20, 21]. If this is generally the case, one is left only with idiotypic suppression as the explanation for the low frequency of these molecules. In any case, these studies of anti-idiotypic antibody structures have provided evidence of yet another mechanism for the generation of antibody diversity.

Summary

For these studies it is clear that within an antigenic system, syngeneic anti-idiotypic antibodies are restricted in their use of germline gene segments. They differ considerably from either allogeneic Ab2s recognizing public idiotopes or syngeneic Ab2s recognizing private idiotopes which are structurally heterogeneous. The D segments of Ab2s in a variety of systems are novel in structure and cannot easily be explained by previously described germline D segments. D-D fusion contributes to the generation of the third hypervariable region in these antibodies. It is not completely clear whether or not this mechanism plays a more important role in generating Ab2s than it does in generating other antibodies. Finally, somatic mutation does occur in anti-idiotypic antibodies. It is unlikely that the idiotypic network, per se, is strictly germline encoded. On the contrary, somatic events (i.e. mutation, junctional diversity, etc.) are probably important in the generation of anti-idiotypic antibodies.

References

1 Jerne, N.K.: Towards a network theory of the immune system. Ann. Immunol. *125:* 373–389 (1974).
2 Kunkel, H.B.; Mannik, M.; Williams, R.C.: Individual antigenic specificity of isolated antibodies. Science *140:* 218–1219 (1963).
3 Oudin, J.; Michel, M.: Une nouvelle forme d'allotypie des globulines gamma du serum lapin apparement liée à la fronction et à la specificité anticorps. C.r. Hebd. séanc. Acad. Sci., Paris *257:* 805–808 (1963).

4 Moser, M.; Leo, O.; Hiernaux, J.; Urbain, J.: Idiotypic manipulations in mice. Balb/c mice can express the cross-reactive idiotype of A/J mice. Proc. natn. Acad. Sci. USA *80:* 4474–4478 (1983).

5 Jerne, N.K.; Roland, J.; Cazenave, P.A.: Recurrent idiotopes and internal images. Eur. molec. biol. Org. J. *1:* 243–247 (1982).

6 Dildrop, R.; Bovens, J.; Siekevitz, M.; Beyreuther, K.; Rajewsky, K.: A V region determinant (idiotope) expressed at high frequency in B lymphocytes is encoded by a large set of antibody structural genes. Eur. molec. biol. Org. J. *3:* 517–523 (1984).

7 Legrain, P.; Rocca-Serra, J.; Moulin, A.; Fougereau, M.; Buttin, G.: A single V_H gene associated with a variety of D and J segments encodes for a large family of ABPC-48-related antibodies induced by anti-idiotypic immunization. Molec. Immunol *22:* 437–443 (1985).

8 Sablitzky, F.; Rajewsky, K.: Molecular basis of an isogenic anti-idiotypic response. Eur. molec. biol. Org. J. *3:* 3005–3012 (1984).

9 Ollier, P.; Rocca-Serra, J.; Somme, G.; Theze, J.; Fougereau, M.: The idiotypic network and the internal image. Possible regulation of a germline network by paucigene encoded Ab2 (anti-idiotypic) antibodies in the GAT system. Eur. molec. biol. Org. J. *4:* 3681–3688 (1985).

10 Bruck, C.; Man, S.C.; Slaoui, M.; Gaulton, G.; Smith, T.; Fields, B.; Mullins, J.; Greene, M.: Nucleic acid sequence of an internal image-bearing monoclonal anti-idiotype and its comparison to the sequence of the external antigen. Proc. natn. Acad. Sci. USA *83:* 6578–6582 (1986).

11 Meek, K.; Jeske, D.; Alkan, S.; Urbain, J.; Capra, J.D.: Structural characterization of syngeneic and allogeneic anti-idiotypic antibodies in the anti-arsonate system. Monogr. Allergy *22:* 109–119 (1987).

12 Meek, K; Capra, J.D.: Stucture and genetics of AB2; in Bona, Biological applications of anti-idiotypes vol. I, pp. 13–21 (CRC Press, Boca Raton 1988).

13 Cheng, H.; Sood, A.K.; Ward, R.E.; Keiber-Emmon, T.; Kohler, H.: Structural basis of stimulatory anti-idiotypic antibodies. Molec. Immunol. *25:* 33–40 (1988).

14 Meek, K.; Hasemann, C.; Pollok, B.; Alkan, S.; Brait, M.; Slaoui, M.; Urbain, J.; Capra, J.D.: Structural characterization of anti-idiotypic antibodies. Evidence that Ab2s are derived from the germline differently than Ab1s. J. exp. Med. *169:* 519–533 (1989).

15 Rajewsky, K.; Takemori, T.: Genetics, expression, and function of idiotypes. An. Rev. Immunol. *1:* 569–607 (1983).

16 Reth, M.; Hammerling, G.J.; Rajewsky, K.: Analysis of the repertoire of anti-NP antibodies in C57B1/6 mice by cell fusion. I. Characterization of antibody families in the primary and hyperimmune response. Eur. J. Immunol. *8:* 393–400 (1978).

17 Kaartinen, M.; Makela, O.: Reading of D genes in variable frames as a source of antibody diversity. Immunol. Today *6:* 324–327 (1985).

18 Rajewsky, K.; Takemori, T.; Reth, M.: In Hammerling, Hammerling, Kearney, Monoclonal antibodies and T cell hybridomas. Perspectives and technical advances, vol. 399 (Elsevier/North-Holland/Biomedical Press, Amsterdam 1981).

19 Wildner, G.: Master's thesis, University of Cologne (1982).

20 Seppalla, J.T.; Eichmann, K.: Induction and characterization of isogeneic anti-idiotypic antibodies to Balb/c myeloma S117. Eur. J. Immunol. *9:* 243–250 (1979).

21 Schuler, W.; Weiler, E.; Kolb, M.: Characterization of syngeneic anti-idiotypic antibody against the idiotype of Balb/c myeloma protein J558. Eur. J. Immunol. *7:* 649–654 (1977).

22 Kurosawa, Y.; Tonegawa, S.: Organization, structure and assembly of immunoglobulin heavy chain diversity DNA segments. J. exp. Med. *155:* 201–218 (1982).

23 Milner, E.C.B.; Meek, K.; Rathbun, G.; Tucker, P.T.; Capra, J.D.: Are anti-arsonate antibody N-segments selected at both the protein and the DNA level? Immunol. Today *7:* 36–39 (1986).

24 Meek, K.; Hasemann, C.; Capra, J.D.: Novel rearrangements at the immunoglobulin D locus. Inversions and fusions add to IgH somatic diversity. J. exp. Med. (in press, 1989).

25 Moser, M.; Leo, O.; Hiernaux, J.; Urbain, J.: Recurrent idiotopes and internal images. Proc. natn. Acad. Sci. USA *80:* 4474–4478 (1963).

26 Alkan, S.: Structural and serological analysis of cross-reactive idiotypes. Comparison of heavy and light chain families of anti-arsonate antibodies. Ann. Immunol., Paris *135c:* 31 (1984).

27 Jeske, D.; Milner, E.C.B.; Leo, O.; Moser, N.; Marver, J.; Urbain, J.; Capra, J.D.: Molecular mapping of idiotopes of anti-arsonate antibodies. J. Immun. *136:* 2568–2574 (1986).

28 Alt, F.W.; Baltimore, D.: Joining of immunoglobulin heavy chain gene segments. Implications from a chromosome with evidence of three D-J_H fusions. Proc. natn. Acad. Sci. USA *79:* 4118–4122 (1982).

29 Rathbun, G.A.; Capra, J.D.; Tucker, P.W.: Organization of the murine immunoglobulin VH complex in the inbred strains. Eur. molec. biol. Org. J. *6:* 2931–2937 (1987).

30 Liu, Z.; Wood, C.; Wu, T.T.: Nucleotide sequence of an anti-fluoroscyl hapten antibody heavy chain variable region gene from a Balb/c mouse hybridoma cell line. Nucl. Acids Res. *15:* 6296 (1987).

31 Kabat, E.A.; Wu, T.T.; Reid-Miller, M.; Perry, H.M.; Gottesman, D.S.: Sequences of proteins of immunologic interest; 4th ed. U.S. Dept. of Health and Human Services, Bethesda, Md. (1987).

32 DNASTAR, Inc., 1801 University Ave., Madison, WI 53705.

33 Sharon, J.; Gefter, M.L.; Manser, T.; Ptashne, M.: Site-directed mutagenesis of an invariant amino acid residue at the variable-diversity segments junction of an antibody. Proc. natn. Acad. Sci. USA *83:* 2628–2631 (1986).

34 Jeske, D.J.; Jarvis, J.; Milstein, C.; Capra, J.D.: Junctional diversity is essential to antibody activity. J. Immun. *133:* 1090–1093 (1984).

35 Legrain, P.; Rocca-Serra, J.; Moulin, A.; Fougereau, M.; Buttin, G.: A single V_H-gene associated with a variety of D and J segments encodes for a large family of ABPC48-related antibodies induced by anti-idiotypic immunization. Molec. Immunol. *22:* 437–443 (1985).

K. Meek, MD, Department of Microbiology, University of Texas Southwestern Medical School, 5323 Harry Hines Blvd., Dallas, TX 75235 (USA)

Carson DA, Chen PP, Kipps TJ (eds): Idiotypes in Biology and Medicine.
Chem Immunol. Basel, Karger, 1990, vol 48, pp 49–62

Patterns of Idiotypic Similarity and Their Structural Bases among Antibodies Specific for Foreign or Self Antigens

F.A. Bonilla, Habib Zaghouani, Constantin Bona

Department of Microbiology, The Mount Sinai School of Medicine of the City University of New York, N.Y., USA

Introduction

Within the past 20 years, large volumes of data have been advanced in support of the notion that recognition of idiotypes of the antigen receptors of B and T cells by self antibodies and lymphocytes plays an important role in the regulation of immune responses [1, 2]. Standing apart from this physiological process of self recognition, however, is the generation of antibodies and lymphocytes in a pathological response to a variety of other self components, resulting in the several autoimmune syndromes. The mechanisms by which tolerance to self antigens is established or lost continue to elude us, and are the focus of a rapidly growing body of literature and speculation. Investigations of idiotypy in autoimmunity are not lacking [2, 3], and the data are consistent with interpretations invoking idiotype-anti-idiotype interactions in autoimmune phenomena.

A number of idiotypic systems have been extensively characterized with respect to antigen specificity, variable region gene usage, suppression or activation by idiotype (Id) or anti-Id, and involvement of Id-specific T cells. The challenge remains, however, to define precisely the structural correlates of immunoglobulin and T cell receptor idiotypes, and, in particular, those structures (if any) which may have a more prominent role than others in determining idiotypic interactions. This latter concept has been termed the 'regulatory idiotope hypothesis' [2, 4].

Regulatory Idiotopes

The regulatory idiotope concept arose from a study of the idiotype of a BALB/c fructan-binding myeloma protein, ABPC48 (A48) [5]. When BALB/c mice are immunized with a fructan such as bacterial levan (BL), less than 10% of the anti-levan antibodies express the A48 idiotype (A48Id). However, when mice are injected at birth with small amounts of A48, or syngeneic polyclonal anti-A48Id antibodies, the anti-BL response generated at age 1 month is 70% A48Id$^+$ [6]. This simple observation led us to examine the processes effecting such a change in the idiotypic character of an immune response.

If we enter the immune network via a single antigen-idiotype pathway, do we encounter endlessly branching paths leading inward, or can we by a short route return to our starting point? Less metaphorically, will an antibody (Ab_1) elicit anti-idiotypic antibodies (Ab_2) reacting only with Ab_1, while Ab_2 elicits anti-Id Ab_3, reacting only with Ab_2, while Ab_3 elicits Ab_4 . . . or, can we detect immunochemical similarities among Ab_1, Ab_2, Ab_3 and Ab_4? This question was addressed in the A48Id system by sequentially immunizing BALB/c mice to produce anti-Id antisera [5]. Mice injected with A48 (Ab_1) produced anti-A48Id antibodies (Ab_2). These Ab_2 were injected to obtain Ab_3 which, in turn, was used to make Ab_4. It was observed that Ab_2 and Ab_4 each react (in a mutually inhibitable fashion) with Ab_3 and Ab_1. Ab_3 differed from Ab_1 in that Ab_3 bound BL very weakly, i.e. BL-binding clones were a minority of those expanded by Ab_2.

The regulatory idiotope hypothesis was advanced to interpret the above findings. Stated simply, not all idiotopes expressed on an immunoglobulin molecule function equally as stimulators or targets of anti-Id antibodies and lymphocytes. From the perspective of the antibodies, this situation may result simply from the frequency with which particular idiotopes are expressed in a given immune response. Only those found in sufficiently high concentration may elicit anti-Id antibodies or T cells. From the point of view of the lymphocytes, preferential recognition of certain idiotopes may result from biases in the repertoire (more frequent paratopes complementary for a given idiotope), or from peculiarities (antigen presentation?) inherent in the response to autologous immunoglobulin.

Thus, immunization with Ab_1 induces the production of Ab_2 recognizing principally the regulatory idiotopes (IdR) of Ab_1. Ab_2 themselves do not express IdR, hence, Ab_3 do not arise by idiotopes of Ab_2 reacting with paratopes of Ab_3, but the opposite: the paratopes of Ab_2 react with idiotopes of Ab_3. Since the combining sites of Ab_2 are directed against IdR, Ab_3 consist mostly of antibodies which express the same IdR as Ab_1. The fact that Ab_3, for the most part, do not share antigen specificity with Ab_1 indicates that a given IdR can be shared by antibodies having a variety of specificities. Since the majority of Ab_3 express the IdR of Ab_1, immunization with Ab_3 produces Ab_4 having much similarity with Ab_2.

Idiotypes Shared by Antibodies with Various Specificities Encoded by Various V Gene Families

The variable regions of A48 and UPC10 (U10), two BALB/c myeloma proteins which bind β (2-6)-fructan (levan), are encoded by genes deriving from the V_HX24 and V_K10 gene families [7–9]. We have analyzed a group of hybridomas obtained from BALB/c mice either treated at birth with A48 or syngeneic polyclonal anti-A48Id antibodies, or adults hyperimmunized with anti-A48Id-KLH conjugates, both groups being challenged with levan 1 month later [10]. These hybridomas were selected for binding to syngeneic polyclonal anti-A48Id antibodies. We found that the majority of these hybridomas reacted to varying degrees with the syngeneic monoclonal anti-A48Id antibody IDA10 [11].

The majority of these A48Id$^+$ monoclonal antibodies (mAbs) use genes deriving from V_HX24 and V_K10 gene families [12, 13]. Analysis of the nucleotide sequences of these genes showed very few somatic mutations in coding regions as compared to germline gene members of the V_HX24 gene family [14], or an A/J germline V_K10 sequence [15], or a BALB/c V_K10 consensus sequence [9]. These results suggested that the A48 regulatory idiotype could be a marker of V_H germline genes since the same V_K10 gene family is used by anti-oxazolone [9], and anti-arsonate [15] antibodies which do not express A48 idiotopes.

We recently studied the binding of IDA10 to a series of A48Id$^+$ proteins in Western blots under reducing and non-reducing conditions [16]. We found that IDA10 does not bind to reduced and separated heavy and light chains, as has been observed in another idiotypic system, where a monoclonal anti-Id specific for PY206 (a BALB/c mAb which binds PR8 influenza virus hemagglutinin) bound to the isolated reduced heavy chain [17]. Thus, it appears that the idiotope recognized by IDA10 is conformational and requires some contribution from the light chain, which either provides proper conformation of the heavy chain and/or contacting residues.

Table 1. V_H genes and specificities represented in 68 monoclonal antibodies assayed for binding to IDA10

V_H	No.	Specificities
7183	24	Br-RBC, CII, DNA, H1, H3, IF, MBP, RF, SA, Sm, Thy, TG
J558	25	α1-3, Dex, Br-RBC, CII, DNA, H1, MBP, NP, RF, Sm, TG
Q52	4	RF, SA, TG
S107	7	H1, NA, PC
J606	5	Br-RBC, INU, Thy
36-60	3	CII, TNP

α1-3 Dex = α1-3 linked dextran; Br-RBC = bromelain-treated mouse red blood cells; CII = collagen type II; H1 and H3 = influenza virus hemagglutinins of PR8 and X31 viruses, respectively; IF = intrinsic factor; INU = inulin; MBP = myelin basic protein; NA = nuclear antigen; NP = (4-hydroxy-3-nitrophenyl)acetyl; PC = phosphorylcholine; RF = rheumatoid factor; SA = skin antigen; Sm = Smith antigen; TG = thyroglobulin; Thy = thymocytes; TNP = trinitrophenyl.

Conformational idiotopes can be expressed by mAbs having similar or different antigen specificities and encoded by V genes from various families. Manheimer-Lory et al. [18] showed that two BALB/c rheumatoid factors, Y19-10 deriving its V genes from V_HJ558 and V_K4 gene families, and 129-48 using V_H7183 (with undetermined V_K gene origin) were both recognized by a polyclonal rabbit anti-Id Fab'$_2$ specific for the LPS10-1 IdX of murine rheumatoid factors [18].

In order to study the expression of the A48Id on antibodies encoded by various gene families, we examined the binding of IDA10 to 70 murine mAbs with various specificities for both exogenous and endogenous antigens [16] (table 1). Among these mAbs, we found five which reacted with IDA10 in a direct-binding solid-phase RIA, in a spot ELISA technique using mAbs bound to nitrocellulose, and in competitive inhibition solid-phase RIA. The characteristics of these mAbs are summarized in table 2. Thus, it appears that antibodies specific for both foreign antigens such as influenza HA, and self antigens such as Sm, can express an A48 idiotope.

Nucleotide sequence analysis of the V genes of these antibodies showed that two mAbs, Z26 and PY102, using genes from V_H7183 and V_K8, while M56 and Y19-10 use genes from V_HJ558 and V_K8 and V_K4, respectively. Therefore, a conformational A48 IdR determinant may be created by V genes deriving from various families. Figure 1 shows a comparison of the

Table 2. Five monoclonal antibodies with different specificities and V genes expressing the A48Id

Name	Origin	Isotype	V_H	V_K	Specificity
M56	LPS-stimulated MRL/lpr splenocytes	IgM	J558	8	Sm
Z26	LPS-stimulated NZB splenocytes	IgM	7183	8	Sm
Y19-10	BALB/c mice immunized with *Yersinia enterocolitica*	IgM	U558	4	RF
PY102	BALB/c mice immunized with PR8 influenza virus	IgG1	7183	8	H1
XY101	BALB/c mice immunized with X31 influenza virus	IgG2b	7182	21	H3

See table 1 for explanations of the abbreviations for antigen specificity. V_H nomenclature is according to Brodeur and Riblet [8]. V_K gene families are numbered according to Potter et al. [29].

amino acid sequences of the V_H regions of A48Id$^+$ antibodies, while figure 2 shows a comparison of the light chain sequences.

We focused our search for homology related to A48Id expression among these sequences by examining the hydrophilicity profiles [19] of the V regions. Amino acid residues which have high hydrophilicity values are predicted to be surface-exposed in solution. This analysis revealed that A48Id$^+$ V regions shared four hydrophilic areas, one in the heavy chain, and three in the light chain (fig. 1, 2).

Kieber-Emmons and Köhler [21] described a 'surface variability analysis' in which a product of the variability (according to Wu and Kabat [20]) and hydrophilicity profiles for a group of sequences highlights areas of the molecule which are both surface-exposed and highly variable. Both of these characteristics make these regions likely places to look for residues contributing to Id expression, hence they were called 'idiotope-defining regions' (IDRs). The homologous and surface-exposed regions of IDA10-reactive mAbs overlap with four of the IDRs (fig. 1, 2).

An examination of V region sequences of antibodies known to be A48Id$^-$ in comparison with those shown in figures 1 and 2 pointed to several residues as having potential idiotope-determining importance. In the heavy chain, 6/6 A48Id$^+$ mAbs have either Asn-Ala or Lys-Ser in positions 73-74, while only 2/11 Id$^-$ sequences have one of these combinations.

```
          1          10          20          30          40          50
          ↓           ↓           ↓           ↓           ↓           ↓
3-14-9    EVKLLESGGGLVQPGGSLNLSCAASGFDFSRYWMSWARQALGKGQEWIGE
ABPC48                                        -----V---P-R-L-----
Z26       --M-----E---K-----K--------T--S-Y-C-XC-TPE-RL-LVAA
M56          Q-APE--K--VPYKM--K---YT-TS-V-H-VK-KPXQXL-X--Y
PY102     --N-V-------K----PK--------T--N-A---V--SPE-RL--VAL
Y19-10    Q-Q-QQP-AK--G--A-VR---K---YT-TG-Y-Y-V--GP-Q-LG---G
```

```
                                       .IDR.D
                              ***************
          a          60          70          80   abc      90
          ↓           ↓           ↓  x++       ↓             ↓
3-14-9    INPGSSTINYTPSLKDKFIISRDNAKNTLYLQMSKVRSEDTALYYC
ABPC48    ---D-----------------------------------------Y
Z26       --S-G-YTY-PDTV-GR-T------R--------SLK---------
M56       ---YNDGT--NEKF-G-ATLTS-KSSS-A-MEL-SLT---S-V---
PY102     -TXXGGNT--PD---GX-T------RDIX-----SL------M---
Y19-10    ----NGGT-FNGRF-GRATLTV-KSSG-A-M-LGGLT-G-S-V---
```

```
          100abcdefghijk              110
          ↓                            ↓
3-14-9    ARLLAK         YAMDYWGQGTSVTVSS    Jh4
ABPC48    -ANWDRGY       WFA------L----A     Jh3
Z26       -SKTGNYYGSS    WYF-V--VX-T-----    JH1
M56       --GNYLA        WFAF-----           Jh3
PY102     G-VRHYG        -G---------X----    Jh4
```

Fig. 1. Comparison of the amino acid sequences of A48Id[+] heavy chains. The row of asterisks indicates an area of hydrophilic residues common to all heavy chains. The letter x indicates residues conserved in the majority of murine V_H regions. A plus sign indicates residues which may be important for A48Id expression. Also indicated is one of the heavy chain idiotope-defining regions (IDR D, see text).

In the light chains, 5/5 Id[+] mAbs have either Arg-Ala or Lys-Ser in positions 24-25, 1/10 Id[-] sequences have Arg-Ala in this location. Five/five Id[+] sequences have Gly or Gln at position 42, 2/6 Id[-] chains have Gln at this position. Finally, 5/5 Id[+] sequences have Gln or Ala and Ile or Leu at positions 80 and 83, respectively. Two/six Id[-] sequences have Ala at 80, and 1/6 has Leu at 83. No Id[-] antibody has all of the residues associated with Id[+] antibodies in all of the surface-exposed areas.

Although particular combinations of residues occur with higher frequency in Id[+] vs. Id[-] sequences, we cannot assume that these residues are all of those which contact the anti-Id, or that they are themselves all contacting residues. The amino acid residues we have focused on may affect idiotope expression by determining the spatial location of residues which may also

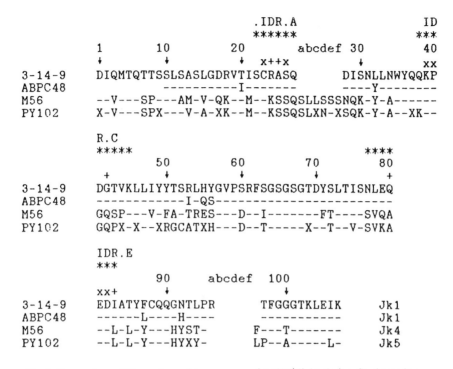

                                        .IDR.A   ID
                                        ******   ***
              1   10   20   abcdef 30   40
              ↓   ↓   ↓   x++x   ↓   xx
3-14-9   DIQMTQTTSSLSASLGDRVTISCRASQ   DISNLLNWYQQKP
ABPC48   ----------I-------   ----Y--------
M56   --V---SP---AM-V-QK--M--KSSQSLLSSSNQK-Y-A------
PY102   X-V---SPX---V-A-XK--M--KSSQSLXN-XSQK-Y-A--XK--

            R.C
            *****
              50   60   70   80
            +   ↓   ↓   ↓   +
3-14-9   DGTVKLLIYYTSRLHYGVPSRFSGSGSGTDYSLTISNLEQ
ABPC48   ------------I-QS--------------------
M56   GQSP---V-FA-TRES---D--I-------FT----SVQA
PY102   GQPX-X--XRGCATXH---D--T-----X--T--V-SVKA

            IDR.E
            ***
              90   abcdef 100
            xx+   ↓   ↓
3-14-9   EDIATYFCQQGNTLPR   TFGGGTKLEIK   Jk1
ABPC48   ------L----H----   -----------   Jk1
M56   --L-L-Y---HYST-   F---T-------   Jk4
PY102   --L-L-Y---HYXY-   LP--A-----L-   Jk5

Fig. 2. Comparison of the amino acid sequences of A48Id[+] light chains. See legend to figure 1 for an explanation of the markings. Also indicated are three idiotope-defining regions (IDRs A, C, and E, see text).

occur in Id⁻ mAbs in positions inappropriate for Id-anti-Id interaction. Experiments utilizing synthetic peptides corresponding to some of these surface-exposed regions in combination with moleclar techniques such as site-directed mutagenesis may permit further elucidation of the structural requirements for IDA10 binding.

Structure of Autoantibody Idiotopes

We have also studied the idiotope expression and V gene usage among 130 self-reactive mAbs [22]. Three idiotypic systems were analyzed: an IdX of anti-DNA antibodies defined by rabbit polyclonal anti-Id antibodies specific for the anti-DNA mAb H130 from the MRL strain [23]; an IdX of anti-Sm antibodies defined by a polyclonal rabbit anti-Id preparation specific for the anti-Sm mAb Y2 from the MRL strain [24], and a rheumatoid factor (RF) IdX defined by polyclonal rabbit anti-Id antibodies against LPS10-1, a BALB/c RF [18].

The data in table 3 show that mAbs derived from various mouse strains with various self reactivities (thyroglobulin, DNA, Sm, collagen type II, intrinsic factor, Fc_γ, skin, microfilaments, and multispecific binding) express one or more of the IdX described above. The most frequent is the LPS10-1 IdX found on 24 self-reactive mAbs. The Y2 and H130 IdXs occurred on 15 and 13 autoantibodies, respectively. Expression of these IdXs does not correlate with the self antigen specificity or the V gene families used by these mAbs.

These observations parallel those described above in the A48Id system. Combinations of V genes different from those expressed in antibodies which define an IdX can generate the IdX. One may envision that such idiotypes may play an important role in the activation of autoreactive clones producing non-organ-specific antibodies through anti-idiotypic interactions.

Expression of Cross-Reactive Idiotypes on Autoantibodies Produced by MRL/lpr Mice Immunized with Foreign Antigen or an Anti-Id Antibody Carrying the Internal Image of the Antigen

In a previous study, we found that 8 of 20 monoclonal autoantibodies from different mouse strains (MRL, SJL, CBA) with various self specificities encoded by genes of the $V_H J558$ gene family also bound to foreign antigens such as glutamic acid-tyrosine (GT) and glutamic acid-phenylalanine (Gl-ϕ) polymers, lysozyme, phenylarsonate, or bacterial polysaccharides. Some of these autoantibodies share the major cross-reactive idiotype of $V_H J558^+$ antibodies specific for foreign antigens [25]. Two of these antibodies express the cGAT IdX [26].

Based on these observations, we studied the frequency of hybridomas producing autoantibodies which bind GT from MRL/lpr mice immunized with GT or an anti-Id antibody (HP20) which bears an internal image of the GT antigen. HP20 has a GTT sequence in the D region; immunization of mice with HP20 elicits antibodies binding GAT and GT [26]. Hybridomas have been prepared from 1-month-old MRL/lpr mice injected at age 2 weeks with GT in FCA, or with either of two anti-Id antibodies (3×50 µg in saline), HP20, or 63-4, an anti-Id against antibodies binding PR8 influenza virus

Table 3. Expression of autoantibody IdXs on self-reactive antibodies encoded by various V_H and V_K genes

Strain	Antibody	Specificity	VH	VK	IdX[a]		
					LPS10-1	Y2	H130
CBA/J	10VA2	TG[b]	J558[c]	1[d]	+	−	+
	84D1	TG	QPC52	8	+	−	−
MRL/lpr	H130	DNA	J558	?	+	−	+
	H241	DNA	J558	4	−	+	+
	Y2	Sm	J558	?	+	+	−
	Y12	Sm	J558	4	+	+	−
	GS13-1	Mult.	S107	1	+	−	−
NZB	CP5	BrMRBC	7083	9	+	−	+
DBA/1	F4	CII	36–60	10	+	−	−
BALB/c	LPS10-1	RF	7183	1	+	−	−
	Y19-10	RF	J558	4	+	+	−
	HB9	MF	7183	1	+	−	−
	HB10	skin	7183	?	+	−	−
	HB12	skin	7183	1	+	−	−
C3H/HeJ	CH46-1	Mult.	J558	22	+	−	−
	CH55-8	Mult.	J558	?	+	−	+
	CH154-1	Mult.	7183	10	+	−	−
	CGS21-7	Mult.	7183	?	−	+	−
C57BL/6	N63-3	Mult.	36-09	19	−	+	+
(nu/nu)	N64-2	TG	S107	10	−	+	−
	N100-1	Mult.	J606	10	+	−	+
me[v]	A23-10	GBM	S107	19	−	+	−
	S2-17-7	Mult.	7183	?	−	+	+
	UN17-19	RF	X24	4	−	+	−
	UN32-15	IF	J558	10	+	−	−
	UN37-5	Mult.	J606	4	−	−	+
	UN40-9	Mult.	7183	1	+	−	+
	UN59-9	Mult.	J558	19	−	+	+

[a] See text for a description of the idiotype systems.

[b] Antigen specificity was studied in solid-phase RIA. TG = Mouse thyroglobulin; DNA = double-stranded DNA; Sm = the nucleoprotein antigen Sm; Mult. = multiple autoantigen reactivity; BrMRBC = bromelain-treated mouse red blood cells; CII = mouse collagen type II; RF = rheumatoid factor; MF = microfibrils; skin = unidentified antigen(s) present in mouse skin; IF = mouse intrinsic factor; GBM = mouse glomerular basement membrane.

[c] V_H gene usage was determined by Northern blotting. Nomenclature is according to Brodeur and Riblet [8].

[d] V_K gene usage was determined by Northern blotting. Numbering is according to Potter et al. [29].

Table 4. Monoclonal antibodies binding GT and/or DNA, Sm, or IgG2a obtained from 1-month-old MRL/lpr mice

Mice injected with	Positive hybridomas/ number screened	Clones obtained
FCA	1/146	FM35-4
GT+FCA	5/694	GP75-9, GP88, GP99-5, GP133, GP138-10
HP20	9/370	H4-2, H8-1, H16-5, H17-1, H45-5, H81-16, H113-1, H127-1, H164-4
63-4	2/120	63-86-7, 63-99-7

FCA = Freund's complete adjuvant.
See text for a description of the idiotype systems.

hemagglutinin. Hybridomas were selected for binding to GT and/or a panel of self antigens (DNA, Sm, and IgG2a) and cloned [22].

Of 694 hybridomas tested from mice immunized with GT, four bind GT and self antigens, only one binds self antigens alone. Of the 370 hybridomas tested from mice immunized with HP20, 8 bind to GT and self antigens, and one to DNA only. Among 120 hybridomas from mice injected with 63-4, only 2 were found to bind DNA. One antibody from mice injected with FCA alone binds DNA (table 4). Table 5 shows the K_d of the binding to GT and self antigens for multispecific antibodies obtained from MRL/lpr mice immunized with GT or anti-Id antibodies. These data show clearly that clones activated by GT or by an antibody carrying an internal image of GT (HP20) synthesize antibodies which have reactivity with self antigens.

We have also studied the expression of four IdXs on these antibodies: the cGAT, LPS10-1, Y2 and H130 IdXs. Table 6 shows the expression of these IdXs on antibodies binding GT and/or self antigens from MRL/lpr mice immunized with GT, or the HP20 or the 63-4 monoclonal anti-Ids.

These data show that the antibodies which bind to GT and self antigens are distinct from the repertoire of antibodies binding GT alone in which the cGAT idiotype is dominant [26]. A minority of these antibodies express the cGAT IdX, while the majority express one or more of the IdXs of anti-DNA, Sm, or RF autoantibodies. Among the multispecific autoantibodies from mice immunized with HP20, some possess the cGAT IdX, while others do not. This agrees with our prediction that an $Ab_{2\beta}$ can stimulate two types of

Table 5. Antigen binding of multispecific antibodies

Antibody	K_d (g/ml $\times 10^8$) with			
	GT	DNA	Sm	IgG2$_a$
GP88	33.3	111	3.70	11.1
GP99-5	6.02	30.8	3.00	46.5
GP133	1.47	1.00	7.50	3.40
GP138-10	270	43.0	39.1	26.0
H4-2	1.02	9.41	65.8	48.1
H8-1	2.24	18.8	–	–
H16-5	4.05	7.08	–	1.79
H45-5	5.65	21.4	75.4	59.5
H113-1	10.5	14.3	–	88.1

– = Not determined.
The K_d was determined in solid-phase RIA according to the method of Friguet et al. [27].

clones: Ag$^+$Id$^+$ and Ag$^+$Id$^-$ by virtue of its mimicry of the antigen [28]. Some cGATId$^-$ clones express autoantibody IdXs.

Conclusion

Altogether, these results show that multispecific clones with binding to foreign and/or self antigens can be activated by immunization with foreign antigens as well as with anti-Id antibodies. Such anti-Id antibodies may be generated in immune responses to foreign antigens and may subsequently lead to activation of autoreactive clones. Clones which originate in responses to foreign antigens may become autoreactive through somatic mutation [30]. Both of these mechanisms may give rise to sharing of idiotopes among antibodies specific for foreign and self antigens.

The findings discussed above indicate clearly that the homologies resulting in idiotype sharing between antibodies do not necessarily correlate with the homologies defining V_H or V_K gene families. Thus, the classical concept that all cross-reactive idiotopes are markers of one or very few V_H or V_K germline genes must be revised. While this may be true for certain particular IdXs, the data indicate that for several of the IdXs we investigated, a fairly large number of germline genes from various gene families may encode the

Table 6. Specificities, V genes and idiotypes of antibodies obtained from 1-month-old MRL/lpr mice

Antibody	Specificity	V_H	V_K	IdX[a]			
				cGAT	LPS10-1	H130	Y2
FM35-4	DNA[b]	J558[c]	4	–	–	–	–
GP75-9	DNA, G2a	J558	8	–	–	–	–
GP88	Mult.	QPC52	9	+	–	–	–
GP99-5	Mult.	7183	1	–	+	+	–
GP133	Mult.	J606	1	–	+	–	–
GP138-10	Mult.	J558	1	–	–	–	–
H4-2	Mult.	J558	9	–	+	–	–
H16-5	Mult.	J558	?	+	+	–	–
H17-1	DNA	QPC52	22	–	–	–	–
H45-5	Mult.	J558	4	+	+	+	–
H81-16	DNA, G2a	QPC52	8		–	–	–
H113-1	Mult.	QPC52	24	+	–	–	–
H127-1	Mult.	QPC52	4	+	–	–	–
H164-4	DNA, GT	QPC52	?	+	–	+	+
63-86-7	DNA	J558	4	–	–	–	–
63-99-7	DNA, G2a	J558	10	–	–	–	–

[a] See text for a description of the idiotype systems.
[b] Antigen specificity was studied in solid-phase RIA. DNA = double-stranded DNA; G2a = murine IgG2a; Mult. = multiple autoantigen binding; GT = glutamic acid-tyrosine polymer.
[c] See table 3 for V_H and V_K gene nomenclature.

particular contacting residues in the particular three-dimensional configuration generating a particular IdX.

These data provide strong experimental support for the concept that autoantibodies and antibodies against foreign antigens may be influenced by similar regulatory processes mediated by idiotypic recognition. These data also suggest that these regulatory processes may contribute to the generation of autoantibody responses and autoimmune disease.

Acknowledgments

This work was supported by National Institute of Allergy and Infectious Diseases Grant No. 1-P01-AI24671, National Science Foundation Grant No. DCB-8790711, and The Council for Tobacco Research USA, Inc. Grant No. 2092R1.

References

1 Jerne, N.K.: Towards a network theory of the immune system. Ann. Immunol., Paris *125C:* 373 (1974).
2 Bona, C.: Regulatory idiotopes (Wiley, New York 1987).
3 Zanetti, M.: Idiotype regulation of autoantibody production. CRC crit. Rev. Immunol. *6:* 151 (1985).
4 Paul, W.E.; Bona, C.: Regulatory idiotypes and immune networks. A hypothesis. Immunol. Today *3:* 230 (1982).
5 Bona, C.A.; Heber-Katz, E.; Paul, W.E.: Idiotype-antiidiotype regulation. I. Immunization with a levan-binding myeloma protein leads to the appearance of auto-anti(anti-idiotype) antibodies and to the activation of silent clones. J. exp. Med. *153:* 951 (1981).
6 Hiernaux, J.; Bona, C.; Baker, P.J.: Neonatal treatment with low doses of anti-idiotypic antibody leads to the expression of a silent clone. J. exp. Med. *153:* 1004 (1981).
7 Auffray, C.; Sikorav, J.L.; Ollo, R.; Rougeon, F.: Correlation between D region structure and antigen-binding specificity. Evidences from the comparison of closely related immunoglobin V_H sequences. Ann. Immunol., Paris *132D:* 77 (1981).
8 Brodeur, P.M.; Riblet, R.: The immunoglobulin heavy chain variable region (Igh-V) locus in the mouse. I. One hundred Igh-V genes comprise seven families of homologous genes. Eur. J. Immunol. *14:* 922 (1984).
9 Legrain, P.; Buttin, G.: The V_K gene expressed by BALB/c ABPC48 cross-reactive idiotypes induced by anti-idiotypic immunization is identical to that of BALB/c anti-oxazolone and A/J anti-arsonate antibodies. J. Immun. *134:* 3468 (1985).
10 Victor-Kobrin, C.; Bonilla, F.A.; Bellon, B.; Bona, C.A.: Immunochemical and molecular characterization of regulatory idiotopes expressed by monoclonal antibodies exhibiting or lacking beta 2-6 fructosan binding activity. J. exp. Med. *162:* 647 (1985).
11 Legrain, P.; Voegle, D.; Buttin, G.; Cazenave, P.-A.: Idiotype-anti-idiotype interactions and the control of the anti-beta(1-6) polyfructosan response in the mouse. Specificity and idiotypy of anti-ABPC48 anti-idiotypic monoclonal antibodies. Eur. J. Immunol. *11:* 678 (1981).
12 Victor-Kobrin, C.; Barak, Z.; Bonilla, F.A.; Bona, C.: Network and regulation of the idiotypic repertoire; in Maurer, Antibodies – structure, synthesis, function and immunologic intervention in disease, p. 91 (Plenum Press, New York 1987).
13 Barak, Z.: Doctoral diss., The City University of New York (1988).
14 Hartman, A.B.; Rudikoff, S.: V_H genes encoding the response to beta(1,6)-galactan. Somatic mutation in IgM molecules. Eur. molec. Biol. Org. J. *3:* 3023 (1984).
15 Meek, K.; Sanz, I.; Rathbun, G.; Nisonoff, A.; Capra, J.D.: Identity of the V_K-Ars-A gene segments of the A/J and BALB/c strains. Proc. natn. Acad. Sci. USA *84:* 6244 (1987).
16 Zaghouani, H.; Bonilla, F.A.; Meek, K.; Bona, C.: Molecular basis for expression of the A48 regulatory idiotope on antibodies encoded by V genes from various families. Proc. natn. Acad. Sci. USA *86:* 2341 (1989).
17 Moran, T.M.; Monestier, M.; Lai, A.C.K.; Norton, G.; Reale, M.A.; Thompson, M.A.; Schulman, J.L.; Riblet, R.; Bona, C.: Characterization of variable region genes and shared cross-reactive idiotypes of antibodies specific for antigens of various influenza viruses. Viral Immunol. *1:* 1 (1987).

18 Manheimer-Lory, A.J.; Monestier, M.; Bellon, B.; Alt, F.W.; Bona, C.A.: Fine specificity, idiotypy and nature of cloned V_H genes of murine monoclonal rheumatoid factor antibodies. Proc. natn. Acad. Sci. USA *83:* 8293 (1986).

19 Hopp, T.P.; Woods, K.R.: Prediction of protein antigenic determinants from amino acid sequences. Proc. natn. Acad. Sci. USA *78:* 3824 (1981).

20 Wu, T.T.; Kabat, E.A.: An analysis of the sequences of the variable regions of Bence-Jones proteins and myeloma light chains and their implications for antibody complementarity. J. exp. Med. *132:* 211 (1970).

21 Kieber-Emmons, T.; Köhler, H.: Towards a unified theory of immunoglobulin structure-function relations. Immunol. Rev. *90:* 29 (1986).

22 Bailey, N.C.; Fidanza, V.; Mayer, R.; Fougereau, M.; Bona, C.: Activation of clones producing self-reactive antibodies by foreign antigen and anti-idiotype antibody carrying the internal image of the antigen. J. clin. Invest. (in press, 1989).

23 Migliorini, P.; Ardman, B.; Kaburaki, J.; Schwartz, R.S.: Parallel sets of autoantibodies in MRL/lpr/lpr mice. An anti-DNA, anti-Sm RNP, anti-gp70 network. J. exp. Med. *165:* 483 (1987).

24 Dang, H.; Fischback, M.; Talal, N.: Anti-idiotypic antiserum to monoclonal anti-Sm inhibits the autoantigen-induced proliferative response. J. Immun. *134:* 3825 (1985).

25 Monestier, M.; Bonin, B.; Migliorini, P.; Dang, H.; Datta, S.; Kuppers, R.; Rose, N.; Maurer, P.; Talal, N.; Bona, C.: Autoantibodies of various specificities encoded by genes from the V_H J558 family bind to foreign antigens and share idiotopes of antibodies specific for self and foreign antigens. J. exp. Med. *166:* 1109 (1987).

26 Mazza, G.; Guigou, V.; Moinier, D.; Corbet, S.; Ollier, P.; Fougereau, M.: Molecular interactions in the GAT idiotypic network. An approach using synthetic peptides. Ann. Immunol., Paris *138:* 3 (1987).

27 Friguet, B.; Chaffotte, A.F.; Djavadi-Ohaniance, L.; Goldberg, M.E.: Measurements of the true affinity constant in solution of antigen-antibody complexes by enzyme-linked immunosorbent assay. J. immunol. Methods *77:* 305 (1985).

28 Bona, C.; Moran, T.: Idiotype vaccines. Ann. Immunol., Paris *136C:* 299 (1985).

29 Potter, M.; Newell, J.B.; Rudikoff, S.; Haber, E.: Classification of mouse V_K groups based on the partial amino acid sequence to the first invariant tryptophan: impact of 14 new sequences from IgG myeloma proteins. Mol. Immunol. *19:* 1619 (1982).

30 Diamond, B.; Scharff, M.D.: Somatic mutation of the T15 heavy chain gives rise to an antibody with autoantibody specificity. Proc. natn. Acad. Sci. USA *81:* 5841 (1984).

F.A. Bonilla, PhD, Department of Microbiology, The Mount Sinai School of Medicine of The City University of New York, New York, NY 10029 (USA)

Carson DA, Chen PP, Kipps T J (eds): Idiotypes in Biology and Medicine.
Chem Immunol. Basel, Karger, 1990, vol 48, pp 63–81

Idiotypic and Molecular Characterization of Human Rheumatoid Factors[1]

Pojen P. Chen, Gregg J. Silverman, Ming-Fei Liu, Dennis A. Carson

Departments of Basic and Clinical Research, Scripps Clinic and
Research Foundation, La Jolla, Calif., USA

Introduction

In most patients with rheumatoid arthritis (RA), their sera contain a
hallmark component, termed rheumatoid factors (RFs) [1–3]. The RFs are
antibody molecules which bind to the Fc region of IgG antibody molecules.
In most rheumatoid patients, their synovial fluid contains abundant aggregates of Ig, which are composed mainly of IgG and RFs. These findings
suggest that RFs may contribute to immune complex formation and chronic
tissue damage in the rheumatoid synovium [2].

Although RFs were originally detected in RA patients, they have also
been found in some patients with other autoimmune diseases including
Sjogren's syndrome (SS), mixed connective tissue disease (MCTD), systemic
lupus erythematosus (SLE), and scleroderma. Furthermore, RFs are found
even in the sera of some apparently normal individuals [1]. For example, IgM
RFs were produced by lymphocytes from normal humans upon in vitro
stimulation with Epstein-Barr virus; and RF precursor cells in normal
subjects increased shortly after a booster immunization with tetanus toxoid
[4]. Similar observations have been made in mice [5–8]. In particular, high
titers of IgM RFs were regularly induced during secondary immune responses in mice. These results suggest that the RF is a physiologic component
of the immune system. Nevertheless, when compared to persons with
nonrheumatoid conditions, the RFs of RA patients are of higher titer, belong

[1] Funding for this research supported in part by grants AR39039, AR33489, and
AR25443 from the National Institutes of Health.

to both IgM and IgG classes, and are produced primarily at extravascular sites [1].

Idiotypes are the serologically defined individual antigenic determinants of antibody molecules. Among them, some are shared by different antibody molecules and are designated cross-reactive idiotypes (CRIs). Analyses of CRIs in 'inbred' mice demonstrate that some CRIs are phenotypic markers for Ig variable region genes (i.e. V_H and V_L) [9–12]. Thus, anti-CRI antibodies have been very useful tools for delineating the genetic basis for murine antibody responses. During the last two decades, we, as well as other investigators, have been applying the same principle to define the genetic components for human RFs. Here, we shall review our current understanding about some well-defined human RF-associated CRIs which have led to the identification of the RF-associated Ig variable region genes.

Idiotypic Characterization of Human Rheumatoid Factors

Analyses with the Classical Polyclonal Anti-Idiotypes

Among human monoclonal IgM RFs derived primarily from individuals with 'mixed cryoglobulinemia', Kunkel et al. [13] used rabbit polyclonal anti-idiotypes to describe two major CRIs, termed Wa and Po. The Wa CRI was expressed by 60% of human monoclonal IgM RFs. Importantly, these authors noted that all Wa-positive RFs contained light chains of the kIIIb sub-subgroup, which constitutes only about 13% of total Ig kappa-chains [14]. Subsequently, Andrews and Capra [15] showed that two Wa-positive RFs were extremely homologous in their light chain variable regions, but not in their heavy chain variable regions. Together, these data suggested strongly that the Wa-CRI is associated mainly with RF light chains.

Analyses with Anti-Idiotypes Induced by Synthetic Hypervariable Region Peptides

Although polyclonal anti-CRI reagents have contributed significantly towards our understanding about the genetic basis of some antibody responses, the genetic meaning of most CRIs are unclear [12]. This may be due to that some polyclonal anti-CRI reagents contain 'homobodies'/'internal image type antiidiotypes' that mimic the three-dimensional structures of antigens, and that most conventional anti-CRI reagents recognize determinants that are dependent on the tertiary and/or quarternary structures of antibody molecules [10, 16–20]. Since Ig heavy and light chain variable region genes are on different chromosomes, genetic studies of CRI defined by the aforementioned reagents require formal breeding experiments, which are not possible in humans.

Thus, in order to lay the ground work for future molecular and genetic studies of human RFs, it was necesary to prepare novel anti-CRI reagents that indentify only the CRIs which depend on the amino acid sequences of either Ig heavy or light chains. Extensive experiments in murine systems have demonstrated that hypervariable regions (complementarity-determining regions, CDRs) are the structural correlates of many idiotypic determinants [10, 11]. In 1983, many investigators had successfully used synthetic peptides to induce antibodies specific for preselected areas in intact proteins [21]. These findings prompted us to use synthetic peptides corresponding to the RF CDRs to generate anti-idiotypes [22–26].

As mentioned earlier, the light chain variable regions of two RFs belonging to the Wa CRI group are remarkably homologous, having identical second CDRs [15]. Accordingly, a PSL2 peptide, corresponding to this CDR and the adjacent framework amino acids, was synthesized and used to immunize rabbits. The resulting anti-PSL2 antiserum bound specifically to the RF Sie and its separated light chains [27]. When nine human monoclonal IgM RFs from patients with mixed cryoglobulinemia were analyzed by immunoblotting, anti-PSL2 antibodies reacted with the separated light chains from 8 of these RFs (fig. 1) [23]. Importantly, antibody binding to these eight RF light chains was completely inhibited by the PSL2 peptide, but not by an unrelated control peptide [23]. These data indicated that the anti-PSL2 antibodies defined an RF light chain-associated CRI.

Thereafter, antibodies were generated against the third CDR of the Sie light chain (PSL3). The anti-PSL3 antisera bound specifically to the intact Sie and the isolated Sie light chains [24]. When the anti-PSL3 antibody was tested against the same nine monoclonal IgM RFs by the immunoblotting method, it reacted with 8 of these RFs (fig. 1) To date, our accumulative data show that anti-PSL2 and anti-PSL3 react, respectively, with about 67 and 57% of human monoclonal IgM RFs from unrelated individuals [3, 25, 28]. It should be noted that most PSL3-positive RFs also express the PSL2-CRI marker.

Are these two CRIs expressed by polyclonal RFs in patients with autoimmune diseases? To this end, sera from individuals with either RA or primary SS were tested. First, the RFs were prepared from plasma by affinity chromatography on a human IgG-coupled Sepharose-4B column. Subsequently, the partially purified autoantibodies were analyzed by immunoblotting. The results showed that anti-PSL2 antibodies reacted with RF light

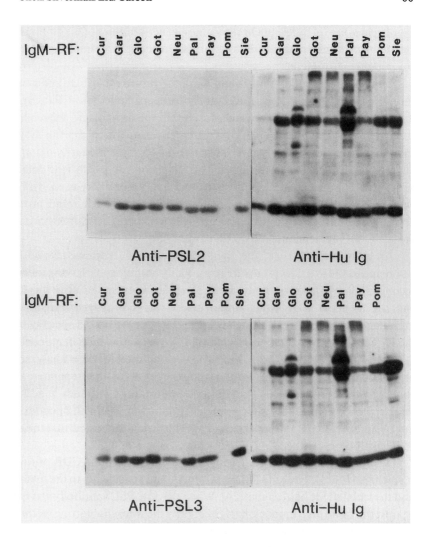

Fig. 1. Immonoblot analyses of nine human monoclonal IgM RFs with the anti-PSL2 and the anti-PSL3 antibodies. About 20 μg of each paraprotein was separated into heavy and light chains by electrophoresis on an SDS-polyacrylamide gel. After transferring to a nitrocellulose paper, the samples were reacted sequentially with the indicated antibodies and then the radiolabeled protein A. After washing, the blot was exposed to XAR film [23, 24, 40].

chains from 5 of 5 RA patients and from 4 of 4 SS patients [29]. Compared to the PSL2-CRI, the PSL3 marker was expressed less frequently. Only 1 of 5 RA patients carried the PSL3-positive RF, compared to 3 of 4 SS patients [29].

Analyses with Monoclonal Anti-Idiotypes

Several investigators have generated murine monoclonal anti-idiotypic antibodies against human RFs. We used a Wa-positive monoclonal RF (Sie) to induce an anti-idiotype, termed 17.109 [30]. The 17.109 antibody reacted efficiently with both intact RF molecules and their separated light chains, and inhibited the binding of RFs to human IgG Fc fragments, indicating that the 17.109 CRI depends mainly on the light chains in the region of the antigen-binding site. It reacted with about 30–50% of monoclonal IgM RFs, including 11/14 Wa-positive monoclonal RFs, but not to any of two Po-positive monoclonal RFs. Importantly, 17.109 bound to a majority of RFs bearing both PSL2 and PSL3 CRIs; and all 17.109-positive RFs were positive for the PSL2-CRI. [25, 28, 29]. As will be discussed later, these three CRIs are related phenotypic markers of a conserved human Vk germline gene, designated Humkv325 [31–33].

When polyclonal RFs were analyzed with this anti-idiotype, 17.109 CRI was detected in sera from most patients with SS and from aged individuals, but not from RA patients [29]. By cytoplasmic staining, 17.109-CRI was found on 2–4% lymphocytes in the salivary tissue of SS patients. In contrast, 17.109 was not detected in rheumatoid synovial membranes [29, 34].

Schrohenloher and Koopman generated a murine monoclonal anti-CRI (designated 6B6.6) from a mouse immunized sequentially with the human monoclonal RFs Cor and Lew [35]. When 50 sera and 20 synovial fluids from seropositive RA patients were analyzed, the 6B6.6 CRI was detected in about one-third of these samples [35]. Subsequently, Crowley et al. [36] analyzed 116 human monoclonal IgMk paraproteins and found that the 6B6.6 CRI was expressed by 7/22 (32%) RFs, but only 3/94 (3%) non-RFs [36]. In addition, they showed that the anti-CRI reacted with the separated light chains of the CRI-positive RFs, suggesting that the 6B6.6 CRI may be the phenotypic marker of a single or a few human Vk genes.

Mageed et al. [37] prepared an anti-CRI antibody (designated G6) from a mouse immunized with a monoclonal IgM RF Kok. They analyzed twelve monoclonal IgM RFs and found five to be positive. In addition, they showed

```
                CRI                           -----CDR1----
            PSL2 PSL3  1                      24    30A  34
Humkv325                EIVLTQSPGT LSLSPGERAT LSCRASQSVS SSYLAWYQQK PGQAPRLLIY
RFs
1-4. CUR,FLO,GAR,GLO
 5.  GOT    ++   ++    ---------- ---------- ---------R ---------- ----------
 6.  PAY    ++   ++    ---------- ---------- ---------- ---------R ----------
 7.  BOR    ++   +     ---------- ---------- ---------- ---------- ----------
 8.  SIE    ++   ++    ---------- ---------- N--------- ----------
 9.  NEU    ++   +     ---------- ---------- -R-------- ----------
10.  WOL    ++   -     ---------- ---------- -G--G----- ----------
11.  KAS    +    ++    D--------- ---------- -------L-  -T-------- ----------
12.  GOL    ++   ++    ---------- ---------- -----ALLS- RG-------- --------M-
Cold agglutinins
 1.  AJ     nd        --------D- ---------- ---------- end of the published seq
 2.  DRE    nd        ---------- ---------- ---------- ------end
 3.  GJ     nd        ---------- --------V- ------end
 4.  MA     nd        ---------- ---------- ---------- end
 5.  NIC    nd        ---------- ---------- ---------- end
 6.  PER    nd        -----Z---- ------Z--- ------Zend
 7   STE    nd        ---------- --------A --end
 8.  TAK    nd        -----Z---- ------Z-V- ---------- ?----end
Anti-LDL antibody
 1.  SON    ++   ++    ---------- ---------- ---------- ---------- ----------
Anti-IF antibody
 1.  PIE    ++   ++    ---------- ---------- ---------- ---------- ----------
Germline Vk genes
 1.  Humkv305         --------A- ---------- ---G------ ---------- --L-------
 2.  Humkv328         ---M----A- --V------- ---------- -N.------- ----------
 3.  Humkv3g          --------A- ---------- ---------- .--------- ----------
 4.  Humkv3g''        --------A- ---------- -------G-- .--------- ----------
 5.  Humkv3h          ---M----P- -------V-- ---------- ----T----- ----------


                       -CDR2--                                   ----CDR3---/
                       50     56                                 89     95 96 Jk
Humkv325                GASSRATGIP DRFSGSGSGT DFTLTISRLE PEDFAVYYCQ QYGSSP
RFs
1-4. CUR,FLO,GAR,GLO                                              R 1, Y 2, Y 2, L 1
         DIFFERENCE
 5.  GOT    1          ---------- ---------- ---------- ---------- ------   R  2
 6.  PAY    1          ---------- ---------- ---------- ---------- ------   L  1
 7.  BOR    2          ---------- ---------- ---------- ----V----- ---N--   Q  1
 8.  SIE    2          ---------- ---------- ---------- -D-------- ------   Q  1
 9.  NEU    4          ---------- ---T------ ------V--- ---------- ---A--   C  2
10.  WOL    4          ---------- ---------- ---------- ---------- ---LG    R  1
11.  KAS    5          --------V- ---------- ---------- ---------- ------   F  4
12.  GOL    7          ---------- ---------- ---------- ---------- ------   R  1
Anti-LDL antibody
 1.  SON    1          ---------- N--------- ---------- ---------- ------   PY 4
Anti-IF antibody
 1.  PIE    0          ---------- ---------- ---------- ---------- ------   W  2
Germline Vk genes
 1.  Humkv305          D--------- ---------- ---------- ---------- ------
 2.  Humkv328          ---T------ A--------- E------S-Q S--------- --NNW-
 3.  Humkv3g           D--N------ A--------- -------S-- ---------- -RSNW-
 4.  Humkv3g''         D--N------ A------P-- -------S-- ---------- -RSNWH
 5.  Humkv3h           ---T---S-- A--------- -------S-Q ---------- -DHNL-
```

that the G6 anti-idiotype reacted with the separated heavy chains of the CRI-positive RFs. Importantly, serological analysis of some G6-positive RFs with Vh subgroup-specific antibodies revealed that all G6-positive RFs contained the Vh1 heavy chains [38].

Molecular Characterization of Human Rheumatoid Factors

Molecular Basis of the PSL2, PSL3 and 17.109 CRIs

In 1984, we noted that the reported amino acid sequence of PSL2-positive RFs were extremely homologous in their variable regions, suggesting that the CRI-positive light chains derived from a single germline gene, designated Vk(RF) [23]. The putative Vk(RF) gene was postulated to encode an amino acid sequence identical to that of the human monoclonal IgM RF Gar. To identify this putative gene, we first screened a human fetal liver genomic library sequentially with a human VkIII cDNA probe NG9/3 and a human VkIII gene probe Humkv301.

Two interesting clones were isolated [31]. Clone 321 contained a partial Vk gene (designated Humkv321). It encodes 54 amino acids, which correspond exactly to the postulated Vk(RF) sequence, from position 42 to 95. Clone 305 contained a Vk gene (designated Humkv305), which shares 92 of 96 amino acids with the postulated Vk(RF) gene. Importantly, Humkv305 and Humkv321 share 300 out of 303 base pairs (bp), and share nine out of ten restriction enzyme sites over a region of 14 kilobases (kb), indicating that these two genes are very homologous [33].

Accordingly, we screened a human placenta DNA library with the Humkv305, and isolated the putative Vk(RF) gene [32, 33]. The cloned Vk

---

Fig. 2. Amino acid sequence comparison of Humkv325 and the kv325-encoded human autoantibodies, including their entire Vk gene encoded regions (positions 1 to 95) and the VJ junctional amino acid residues [3, 15, 28, 31–33, 39–42, 46]. The Jk gene usage is indicated and the PSL2 and PSL3 CRI expression of these autoantibodies are given. The deduced amino acid sequence of Humkv325 is given at the top. All the other sequences are first aligned for maximum homology, and the residues identical to kv325 are indicated by bars whereas the introduced gaps are marked by dots. The numbers after each autoantibody denote the number of residues by which the respective sequence deviates from kv325 sequence. All other human functional VkIII germline genes are included to show that they are unlikely to encode any of the PSL2-positive RF light chains. Humkv3g, Humkv3g'' and Humkv3h are renamed from the Vg, Vg'' and Vh genes reported previously [46].

gene, designated Humkv325, encodes exactly the 96 amino acid residues of the RF Gar sequences, and is identical to Humkv321 in the overlapped area, indicating that Humkv325 is the full-length gene for Humkv321.

To date, the amino acid sequences of 12 PSL2-positive light chains have been determined [15, 39–42]. When these sequences were compared with the Humkv325 sequence, four are identical to Humkv325. The remaining 8 differ from the Humkv325 by 1–7 amino acid residues only (fig. 2). Regarding the Jk gene usage, Humkv325 can be joined to Jk1, Jk2 or Jk4 gene segments to generate RF light chains. The VJ rearrangement results in different junctional amino acid residues for Jk1 and Jk2 (i.e. R, L, Q, and Y, R, C, respectively). Collectively, these data demonstrate that a human Vk gene can encode RF light chains either with or without somatic changes, and that the Humkv325 exists widely among outbred populations, including normal subjects, as well as patients with autoimmune diseases.

Molecular Basis of the 6B6.6 CRI

Among 6B6.6-positive RF light chains, we noted that the amino acid sequences of Cla, Pom and Les were homologous (fig. 3) [43, 44]. In addition, a comparison of the deduced amino acid sequence of all isolated human VkIII germline genes with the reported amino acid sequences of all human VkIII light chains suggested that at least one additional VkIII gene exists in the germline, which encodes Cla, Les, Pom and other VkIII light chains [33, 45, 46]. Most of these light chains have characteristic amino acids at positions 4 (Met), 9 (Ala), 13 (Val) and a deletion of Tyr at position 32.

To isolate this putative RF-associated Vk gene, a genomic DNA library from the patient Les was screened with the rearranged Les light chain gene, and positive clones were characterized. One new Vk gene, designated Humkv328, was isolated [47].

As can be seen in figure 3, kv328 is most closely related to the Les light chain, differing from Les by only 3 among a total of 95 residues [44, 47]. To examine this further, we sequenced an additional 633 bp upstream of ka3les (from −904 to −272), and compared the ka3les sequence with the kv328 sequence. The result showed that Humkv328 shared with ka3les 1315/1331 nucleotides at the DNA level, and 109/112 amino acid residues at the protein level (including the leader peptide) [48]. Importantly, kv328 shares with Les the distinct characteristics of having Val (instead of Leu) at the position 13, and of lacking Tyr at the position 32 in the first CDR. The relatively conserved Leu and Tyr residues are present in most reported VkIII light

```
          6B6.6 CRI                              -----CDR1----
RFs                 1                       24     30A   34                    49
1. LES      +       EIVMTQSPAT LSVSPGERAT LSCRASQSVS NN.LAWYQQK PGQPPRLLIY
2. POM      +       --------V- ---------- --------I- -SY------- -SGS------
3. CLA      +       ---------- ---------- ------end of the published sequence
4. SHE      nd      ---------- ---------- ---end
Germline Vk genes
            DIFFERENCE
Humkv328    3       ---------- ---------- ---------- S--------- ---A------
Humkv3g     12      ---L------ --L------- ---------- .SY------- ---A------
Humkv3h     14      --------P- --L-----V- ---------- SSY-T----- ---A------
Humkv325    14      ---L----G- --L------- ---------- SSY------- ---A------
Humkv3g''   15      ---L------ --L------- -------G-- .SY------- ---A------
Humkv305    16      ---L------ --L------- ---G------ SSY------- --LA------


                    -CDR2--                               ----CDR3
RFs                 50     56                            89         95
1. LES              GASTRATGIP ARFSGSGSGT EFTLTISRLQ SEDFAVYYCQ QYNNWP
2. POM              ---------- ---------- -------S-- ---------- ------
Gerline Vk genes
Humkv328            ---------- ---------- -------S-- ---------- ------
Humkv3g             D--N------ ---------- D------S-E P--------- -RS---
Humkv3h             -------S-- ---------- D------S-- P--------- -DH-L-
Humkv325            ---S------ D--------- D--------E P--------- --GSS-
Humkv3g''           D--N------ -------P-- D------S-E P--------- -RS--H
Humkv305            D--S------ D--------- D--------E P--------- --GSS-
```

Fig. 3. Amino acid sequence comparison of the 6B6.6 positive RF light chains and Humkv328, as well as all reported human functional VkIII germline genesequences [43–45]. The residues at position 9 of the Cla and She were determined to be both Ala and Gly [45]. The complete sequence of the RF Les light chain is given. All the other sequences are first aligned for maxium homology, and the residues identical to Les are indicated by bars whereas the introduced gaps are marked by dots. The numbers after each sequence denote the number of residues by which the respective sequence differs from the Les sequence. All other human functional VkIII germline genes are included to show that they are unlikely to encode any of the 6B6.6-positive RF light chains. Humkv3g, Humkv3g'' and Humkv3h are renamed from the Vg, Vg'' and Vh genes reported previously [46].

chain protein sequences and in all functional VkIII germline genes that have been sequenced previously. Besides, Hmkv328 is identical to the Pom light chain from positions 44 to 95, and to the sequences of RFs Cla and She from positions 1 to 23/26. Together, these data strongly suggest that kv328 is the corresponding germline gene for the rearranged Les light chain gene, as well as three other RF light chains; and that Humkv328 may be the genetic basis for the 6B6.6 CRI in humans.

Molecular Basis of the G6 CRI

Recently, Capra and colleagues found that the heavy chains of two G6-positive RFs (i.e. Bor and Kas) shared an 86% homology from residues 1 to 94, corresponding to the Vh encoded region (fig. 4) [42]. In addition, they noted that these two RF Vh sequences were most homologous to a rearranged Vh gene, termed 783 [communiated to Newkirk et al., 42, by Ravetch and Korsmeyer]. In addition, we noted that a Vh1 cDNA clone 51P1 differed from Bor and Kas by only 8 residues each (fig. 4) [49–52]. Accordingly, we screened a human genomic library separately with both 783 and 51P1, and the strongly positive clones were isolated and characterized by restriction mapping and sequence analysis. The results show that one isolate contains a human Vh1 gene, designated Humhv1263, which is highly homologous to 51P1, and to 783 in the coding region, but not in the 5′ flanking region [53].

The 783 gene was only mentioned by Newkirk at al. [42] in a comparison of RF heavy chains with some human Vh1 sequences [42]. This Vh gene was isolated from a chronic lymphocytic leukemia (CLL), termed LR35 [54; Korsmeyer, personal commun.], and its DNA sequence (designated Humighaa) was deposited by Ravetch and Leder in GenBank. As mentioned earlier, Humhv1263 is highly homologous to Humighaa in the coding region, but not in the upstream flanking region. The result suggested that there may be some sequence errors in the deposited sequence of Humighaa. Accordingly, we resequenced a 366-bp fragment (BamH1-BamH1) of the 783/Humighaa gene. We found that our DNA sequence of 783 differs from the deposited 783 sequence by 27 bases, and that the revised 783 sequence is identical to the 51P1 sequence, except one difference near the VD junction [53]. Since 783 and 51P1 were isolated from two unrelated individuals [49, 54], these results strongly indicate that, up to the A nucleotide at the amino acid position 98, the 783 sequence is likely to be the unmutated form of its corresponding germline Vh gene.

When the deduced amino acid sequences of hv1263, 783 and all other reported human Vh1 genes were compared with the heavy chains of RFs Bor and Kas, 783c is the most closely related one. It differs from Kas and Bor by only 7 and 9 residues, respectively (fig. 4). In contrast, germline gene hv1263 differs from Kas and Bor by 11 and 12 residues, respectively; while all other Vh1 germline genes each differ from both RFs by 22–40 residues (fig. 4). Detailed molecular analyses of CRIs in mice reveal that variant antibody molecules deviate from their respective germline genes by up to 8 amino acid residues, and that the extent of somatic diversifications on the heavy chain and light chain of a variant antibody molecule are correlated to each other

```
              DIFFERENCE                                  CDR 1               CDR2
RFs              1                                      31--35               50-
1. BOR          <EVQLVQSGAE VKKPGSSVKV TCKASGDTFS SSAISWVRQA PGQGLEWMGG
2. KAS     13    --H------- ---------- S-----G--- -Y-------- ----------
3. SIE     40    ---------- --------R- ---T--G--- GYT------- --R----V-S
4. WOL     41    ----M----- --------R- S--T--G--V DYKGL----- --K----V-Q
Vh cDNA
1. 51P1     8    Q--------- ---------- S-----G--- -Y-------- ----------
Rearranged Vh gene
1. 783      9    Q--------- ---------- S-----G--- -Y-------- ----------
Germline Vh genes
1. hvl263  12    Q--------- ---------- S-----G--- -Y-------- ---------R
2. 21-2    22    Q--------- -----A---- S-----Y--T -YYMH----- ---------I
3. HG3     22    Q--------- -----A---- S-----Y--N -YYMH----- ---------I
4. 7-2     24    QM-------- ---T------ S-----Y--T YRYLH----- ---A-----W
Germline pseudogenes
1. V71-5   25    QM------P- -----T---- S-----F--T ---VQ----- R--R---I-W
2. 1-1     26    Q--------- ---L-A---- S-----Y--T GYYMH--X-- ---------W
3. HA2     28    Q----*---- -----A---- S-----Y--T -YYMN-M--- ----F----W
4. 8-2     32    Q-------D- M--A-A---- S--TC-Y--T -YSMH*---- HA-------R
5. V201    38    Q---L-P-VQ ---------- S-*--RY--T KYFTR--*-S ----HX---*


                 CDR2
RFs              ---------------66                                         98
1. BOR           IIPIFGTPNY AQKFQGRVTI TTDESTSTAY MEVSSLRSED TALYYCAR
2. KAS           ------QA-- ---------- -A----N--- --LR----D- --M----K
3. SIE           PAKWTDPFQG VYIKWE---V SLKP-FNQ-- --LVN-FN-- G-V-----
4. WOL           -PLR-NGEVK NPGSVV--SV SLKP-FNQ-H --L---F--- --V-----
Vh cDNA
1. 51P1          -------A-- ---------- -A-------- --L------- --V-----
Rearranged Vh gene
1. 783           -------A-- ---------- -A-------- --L------- --V----K
Germline Vh genes
1. hvl263        ----L-IA-- ---------- -A-K------ --L------- --V-----
2. 21-2          -N-SG-STS- ---------M -R-T----V- --L------- --V-----
3. HG3           -N-SG-STS- ---------M -R-T----V- --L------- --V-----
4. 7-2           -T-FN-NT-- -----D---- -R-R-M---- --L------- --M-----
Germline pseudogenes
1. V71-5         -VVGS-NT-- -----E---- -R-M------ --L------- --V----A
2. 1-1           -N-NS-GT-- ---------M -R-T-I---- --L-R---D- --V-----
3. HA2           -NAGN-NTK- S--L------ -R-T-A---- -QL------- --V-----
4. 8-2           MC-SD-SIS- -E-------M -R-T------ --L------- --M---G-
5. V201          -N-YNDNTH- --T-W----- -S-R-M---- --L-X----- MVV---V-
```

Fig. 4. Amino acid sequence comparison of four Wa- and G6-positive RF heavy chains (Bor, Kas, Sie and Wol), one Vh1 cDNA (51P1), one Vh1 rearranged gene (783) and all available sequenced human Vh1 germline genes [15, 42, 49, 50–54]. The Bor heavy chain sequence is given at the top. All the other sequences are first aligned for maxium homology, and the residues identical to Bor are indicated by bars whereas the introduced gaps are marked by dots. The numbers after each sequence denote the number of amino acid residues in which the respective sequence deviates from RF Bor heavy chain.

[55–57]. The latter phenomena are called 'parallel diversifications'. A comparison of Bor and Kas light chains with all human Vk germline genes shows that both are encoded by Humkv325 with 2 and 5 amino acid substitutions, respectively. Combined, these data suggest that the putative '783 Vh gene' is likely to encode the heavy chains of RFs Bor and Kas.

Since both RFs Bor and Kas are positive for the G6 CRI, it appears that the 783 Vh gene may be the genetic basis for the G6 CRI. However, it should be noted that RFs Sie and Wol also bear the G6 CRI, and their heavy chain variable regions differ extensively from Bor, Kas and 783 (fig. 4). Accordingly, more G6-positive heavy chains should be sequenced in order to define the structural correlates of the G6 CRI.

Discussion

An idiotype is an antigenic determinant of an antibody variable region. It is now well established that some CRIs are the phenotypic markers of the Ig V genes, while most private idiotypes are the results of somatic mutations. As reviewed here, idiotypic analyses of human monoclonal RFs derived mainly from individuals with cryogobulinemia showed that there were some major RF-associated CRIs, and subsequent molecular studies of these CRIs revealed that they represent the phenotypic markers of some human Ig V genes. In addition to monoclonal RFs, some of these RF-associated CRIs are also expressed by polyclonal RFs in patients with RA and primary SS. Collectively, these data indicate that human RFs are heterogenous, and utilize several Ig V genes which are widely distributed among outbred human populations.

It has been shown that some idiotypes were shared by antibodies which had different specificities [58, 59]. These data suggested that antibodies of different specificities might be encoded by the same Ig V genes for either their light chains or heavy chains [10, 12]. In humans, we noted that the Humkv325 sequence is identical to the light chain variable region of an autoantibody (Pie) against intermediate filament (IF), and differs by only one amino acid residue from the light chain variable region of an autoantibody (Son) against low-density lipoprotein (LDL) (fig. 2) [39]. As expected, both Son and Pie are positive for the PSL2 and PSL3 CRIs. Using the same anti-idiotypes, Agnello et al. [60] found that two cold agglutinins (i.e. Gag and Joh) expressed the PSL2 CRI [60]. Similarly, we found that anti-PSL2 antibodies reacted with 6/6 cold agglutinins, while anti-PSL3 antibodies reacted with only 3/6 cold agglutinins. These observations were consistent with the partial amino acid sequence analyses of 7 cold agglutinins (i.e. MA, NIC, DRE, PER, STE, GJ, TAK; from position 1 to position 22) which contained the diagnostic amino acid residues of the Humkv325 gene (i.e. Leu, Gly and Leu at positions 4, 9, and 13, respectively) (fig. 2) [46]. In addition to autoantibodies, we recently found that both PSL2 and PSL3 CRIs were expressed by a human monoclonal anti-CMV antibody (Ev), suggesting that the antivirus antibody used the Humkv325 gene for its light chain. This conclusion was indeed supported by the amino acid sequence of the Ev ligh chain [61]. Combined, these data demonstrate that the Humkv325 is frequently used by autoantibodies of various specificities, and, to a lesser degree, by antibodies to foreign antigens.

Recently, we noted that Humkv325 may encode the great majority of the reported VkIII light chains [33]. Among 20 complete VkIII light chain sequences (B6, Bor, Cur, Flo, Fr4, Gar, Glo, Gol, Got, Kas, Les, Neu, Pay, Pie, Pom, Sie, Son, Ti, V41 and Wol), 18 probably derive from kv325. Furthermore, among 58 other partial VkIII light chain sequences, at least 19 are probably encoded by the kv325 gene. In addition, it was found that approximately 20% of CLL bore the 17.109 CRI, and that all CRI-positive CLL expressed the Humkv325 gene [62, 63]. As described earlier, the kv325-encoded light chains have been associated with autoantibodies against IgG, LDL, IF and erythrocytes. Recently, data from human and murine systems suggested that autoreactive B cell precursors are often in a proliferative state [64–66]. Accordingly, it is conceivable that B cells expressing the kv325 gene are likely to react with self components, and thus may be stimulated by autoantigens to proliferate constantly. The continual cell cycling would render the kv325-bearing cells exceptionally susceptible to abnormal clonal expansion and malignant transformation. If substantiated, this hypothesis may explain why the kv325 gene is expressed by a large proportion of CLL, and are overly represented among Ig paraproteins and/or Bence-Jones light chains.

In contrast to the recurrent 'sequence-dependent' CRIs on RF light chains, the idiotypes on the RF heavy chains appeared to be more individually specific. Six peptides were synthesized, corresponding to the second and the third heavy chain CDRs of the RFs Sie, Wol and Pom. Among the six corresponding antipeptide antisera, five reacted specifically with the appropriate parental protein [24]. When a total of 24–25 IgM RFs were analyzed by immunoblotting, all antipeptide antibodies reacted only with the corresponding parental proteins, except for anti-PSH3, which bound to two additional RFs [24, 25, 42]. These results suggest either that RF heavy chains are encoded by a number of different Vh and Dh genes, or that human monoclonal RF heavy chains display an unusually high degree of somatic mutation in a restricted number of Vh genes, as well as significant variation in VDJ gene joining.

To further define the heavy chain components of human monoclonal IgM RFs, we synthesized three different peptides corresponding to the diagnostic amino acid residues in the first framework regions of all three human heavy chain subgroups, and used them to induce sequence-dependent heavy chain subgroup-specific antibodies. When a total of 25 human monoclonal RFs were analyzed, 14, 3, and 8 RFs have $V_H I$, II, III heavy chains, respectively [38]. Importantly, 13/14 and 9/14 $V_H I$ RFs bear the PSL2 and 17.109 CRIs, respectively. On the other hand, anti-$V_H I$ antibodies reacted with 13/17 PSL2-positive RFs and 10/14 17.109-positive RFs. Among the remaining 4 PSL2- and 17.109-positive RFs, 2 contained $V_H II$ heavy chains, while another 2 had $V_H III$ heavy chains. Together, these results demonstrated that the Humkv325-encoded RFs preferentially, but not exclusively, used the $V_H I$ heavy chain genes; and that the majority of the $V_H I$ gene-encoded RFs employed the Humkv325 gene. In contrast, one kv328-encoded RF (Les) contained the $V_H II$ heavy chain, while the other one kv328-encoded RF (Pom) had the $V_H III$ heavy chain. Similar results had been observed in studies of murine monoclonal RFs [67, 68].

Usually, during an antigen-driven immune response, antibodies with higher affinities, that have been generated via a process of random somatic mutations, are selected and expanded, and become the dominant antibody species [69]. On the contrary, without a selection pressure, the germline-encoded antibodies are the dominant antibody species. As described earlier, PSL2, PSL3 and 17.109 CRIs were expressed by a significant portion of RFs from patients with cryoglobulinemia and SS, but not patients with RA. These data suggest that continued RF synthesis in RA patients is driven by a conventional antigen, while RF production in patients with cryoglobulinemia and SS is at least partly the consequence of an antigen-independent proliferation of autoreactive B cell clones. In this regard, clinical data showed that 10/30 of the patients with primary SS had mixed monoclonal IgM cryoglobulins, and that 3/58 of the patients with SS developed reticulum cell sarcoma [70, 71].

In summary, following the lead from idiotypic studies of human RFs, we have identified two RF-associated Vk genes and one RF-associated Vh gene.

With these Ig V gene probes, we can now assess the polymorphisms of RF-related V genes in humans and their role in the genetic aspect of human autoimmune diseases.

Acknowledgments

We thank Drs. J.D. Capra, J.J. Crowley, S. Fong, Blas Frangione, F. Goni, T.J. Kipps, W.J. Koopman, R. Jefferis, R.A. Mageed, and R.E. Schrohenloher for their significant contributions toward our collaborative studies of human RFs. We acknowledge the excellent technical assitance of S. Sinha, and the secretarial assistance of Ms. Jane Uhle and the BCR Word Processing Center in the preparation of this manuscript.

References

1 Carson, D.A.; Chen, P.P.; Fox, R.I.; et al.: Rheumatoid factors and immune networks. A. Rev. Immunol. *5:* 109–126 (1987).

2 Carson, D.A.: Rheumatoid factor; in Kelley, Harris, Ruddy, et al., Textbook of rheumatology, pp. 664–676 (Saunders, Philadelphia 1985).

3 Chen, P.P.; Fong, S.; Carson, D.A.: Rheumatoid factor. Rheum. Dis. N. Am. *13:* 545–568 (1987).

4 Welch, M.J.; Fong, S.; Vaughan, J.H.; et al.: Increased frequency of rheumatoid factor precursor B lymphocytes after immunization of normal adults with tetanus toxoid. Clin. exp. Immunol. *51:* 299–305 (1983).

5 Coulie, P.; Van Snick, J.: Rheumatoid factors and secondary immune responses in the mouse. II. Incidence, kinetics and induction mechanisms. Eur. J. Immunol. *13:* 895–899 (1983).

6 Coulie, P.G.; Van Snick, J.: Rheumatoid factor (RF) production during anamnestic immune responses in the mouse. III. Activation of RF precursor cells is induced by their interaction with immune complexes and carrier-specific helper T cells. J. exp. Med. *161:* 88–97 (1985).

7 Nemazee, D.A.; Sato, V.L.: Induction of rheumatoid antibodies in the mouse: regulated production of autoantibody in the mouse: regulated production of autoantibody in the secondary humoral response. J. exp. Med. *158:* 529–545 (1983).

8 Nemazee, D.A.: Immune complexes can trigger specific, T cell-dependent, autoanti-IgG antibody production in mice. J. exp. Med. *161:* 242–256 (1985).

9 Weigert, M.; Riblet, R.: The genetic control of antibody variable regions in the mouse. Springer Semin. Immunopathol. *1:* 133–169 (1978).

10 Rajewsky, K.; Takemori, T.: Genetics, expression, and function of idiotypes. An. Rev. Immunol. *1:* 569–607 (1983).

11 Rudikoff, S.: Immunoglobulin structure-function correlates. Antigen binding and idiotypes. Contemp. Top. mol. Immunol. *9:* 169–209 (1983).

12 Capra, J.D.; Fougereau, M.: Structural correlates of idiotypes. One from column A, one from column B. Immunol. Today *4:* 177–179 (1983).

13   Kunkel, H.G.; Agnello, V.; Joslin, F.G.; et al.: Cross-idiotypic specificity among monoclonal IgM proteins with anti-gammaglobulin activity. J. exp. Med. *137:* 331–342 (1973).

14   Kunkel, H.G.; Winchester, R.J.; Joslin, F.G.; et al.: Similarities in the light chains of anti-gamma-globulins showing cross-idiotypic specificities. J. exp. Med. *139:* 128–136 (1974).

15   Andrews, D.W.; Capra, J.D.: Complete amino acid sequence of variable domains from two monoclonal human anti-gamma globulins of the Wa cross-idiotypic group. Suggestion that the J segments are involved in the structural correlate of the idiotype. Proc. natn. Acad. Sci. USA *78:* 3799–3803 (1981).

16   Lindenmann, J.: Speculation on idiotypes and homobodies. Ann. Immunol., Paris *124C:* 171–222 (1973).

17   Jerne, N.K.: Towards a network theory of the immune system. Ann. Immunol., Paris *125C:* 373 (1974).

18   Nisonoff, A.; Lamoyi, E.: Implications of the presence of an internal image of the antigen in anti-idiotypic antibodies. Possible application to vaccine production. Clin. Immunol. Immunopathol. *21:* 397–406 (1981).

19   Jerne, N.K.; Roland, J.; Cazenave, P-A.: Recurrent idiotypes and internal images. Eur. molec. Biol. org. J. *1:* 243–247 (1982).

20   Kohler, H.; Muller, S.; Bona, C.: Internal antigen and immune network. Proc. Soc. exp. Biol. Med. *178:* 189–195 (1985).

21   Lerner, R.A.: Antibodies of predetermined specificity in biology and medicine. Adv. Immunol. *36:* 1–44 (1984).

22   Chen, P.P.; Houghten, R.A.; Fong, S.; et al: Anti-hypervariable region antibody induced by a defined peptide. An approach for studying the structural correlates of idiotypes. Proc. natn. Acad. Sci. USA *81:* 1784–1788 (1984).

23   Chen, P.P.; Goni, F.; Fong, S.; et al.: The majority of human monoclonal IgM rheumatoid factors express a 'primary structure-dependent' cross-reactive idiotype. J. Immun. *134:* 3281–3285 (1985).

24   Chen, P.P.; Goni, F.; Houghten, R.A.; et al.: Characterization of human rheumatoid factors with seven antiidiotypes induced by synthetic hypervariable region peptides. J. exp. Med. *162:* 487–500 (1985).

25   Chen, P.P.; Fong, S.; Goni, F.; et al.: Analyses of human rheumatoid factors with antiidiotypes induced by synthetic peptides. Monogr. Allergy *22:* 12–23 (1987).

26   Chen, P.P.; Fong, S.; Carson, D.A.: The use of defined peptides in characterizing idiotypes. Int. Rev. Immunol. *2:* 419–432 (1987).

27   Chen, P.P.; Fong, S.; Normansell, D.; et al.: Delineation of a cross-reactive idiotype on human autoantibodies with antibody against a synthetic peptide. J. exp. Med. *159:* 1502–1511 (1984).

28   Chen, P.P.; Fong, S.; Goni, F.; et al.: Cross-reacting idiotypes on cryoprecipitating rheumatoid factor. Springer Semin. Immunopathol. *10:* 35–55 (1988).

29   Fong, S.; Chen, P.P.; Gilbertson, T.A.; et al.: Expression of three cross reactive idiotypes on rheumatoid factor autoantibodies from patients with autoimmune diseases and seropositive adults. J. Immun. *137:* 122–128 (1986).

30   Carson, D.A.; Fong, S.: A common idiotype on human rheumatoid factors identified by a hybridoma antibody. Mol. Immunol. *20:* 1081–1087 (1983).

31   Chen, P.P.; Albrandt, K.; Orida, N.K.; et al.: Genetic basis for the cross-reactive idiotypes on the light chains of human IgM anti-IgG autoantibodies. Proc. natn. Acad. Sci. USA *83:* 8318–8322 (1986).

32 Radoux, V.; Chen, P.P.; Sorge, J.A.; et al.: A conserved human germline Vk gene directly encodes rheumatoid factor light chains. J. exp. Med. *164:* 2119–2124 (1986).

33 Chen, P.P.; Albrandt, K.; Kipps, T.J.; et al.: Isolation and characterization of human VkIII germline genes. Implications for the molecular basis of human VkIII light chain diversity. J. Immun. *139:* 1727–1733 (1987).

34 Fox, R.I.; Chen, P.P.; Carson, D.A.; et al.: Expression of a cross reactive idiotype on rheumatoid factor in patients with Sjogren's syndrome. J. Immun. *136:* 477–483 (1986).

35 Schrohenloher, R.E.; Koopman, W.J.: An idiotype common to rheumatoid factors from patients with rheumatoid arthritis identified by a monoclonal antibody. Arthritis Rheum. *29:* S28 (1986).

36 Crowley, J.J.; Goldfien, R.D.; Schrohenloher, R.E.; et al.: Incidence of three cross-reactive idiotypes on human rheumatoid factor paraproteins. J. Immun. *140:* 3411–3418 (1988).

37 Mageed, R.A.; Dearlove, M.; Goodall, D.M.; et al.: Immunogenic and antigenic epitopes of immunoglobulins. XVII. Monoclonal anti-idiotypes to the heavy chain of human rheumatoid factors. Rheumatol. int. *6:* 179–183 (1986).

38 Silverman, G.J.; Goldfien, R.D.; Chen, P.; et al.: Idiotypic and subgroup analysis of human monoclonal rheumatoid factors. Implications for structural and genetic basis of autoantibodies in humans. J. clin. Invest. *82:* 469–475 (1988).

39 Pons-Estel, B.; Goni, F.; Solomon, A.; et al.: Sequence similarities among kIIIb chains of monoclonal human IgMk autoantibodies. J. exp. Med. *160:* 893–904 (1984).

40 Goni, F.; Chen, P.P.; Pons-Estel, B.; et al.: Sequence similarities and cross-idiotypic specificity of L chains among human monoclonal IgM-K with anti-gammaglobulin activity. J. Immun. *135:* 4073–4079 (1985).

41 Newkirk, M.; Chen, P.P.; Carson, D.A.; et al.: Amino acid sequence of a light chain variable region of a human rheumatoid factor of the Wa idiotypic group, in part predicted by its reactivity with antipeptide antibodies. Mol. Immunol. *23:* 239–244 (1986).

42 Newkirk, M.M.; Mageed, R.A.; Jefferis, R.; et al.: Complete amino acid sequences of variable regions of two human IgM rheumatoid factors, BOR and KAS of the Wa idiotypic family, reveal restricted use of heavy and light chain variable and joining region gene segments. J. exp. Med. *166:* 550–564 (1987).

43 Capra, J.D.; Klapper, D.G.: Complete amino acid sequence of the variable domains of two human IgM anti-gamma globulins (Lay/Pom) with shared idiotypic specificities. Scand. J. Immunol. *5:* 677–684 (1976).

44 Jirik, F.R.; Sorge, J.; Fong, S.; et al.: Cloning and sequence determination of a human rheumatoid factor light-chain gene. Proc. natn. Acad. Sci. USA *83:* 2195–2199 (1986).

45 Ledford, D.K.; Goni, F.; Pizzolato, M.; et al.: Preferential association of kappa-IIIb light chains with monoclonal human IgM-kappa autoantibodies. J. Immun. *131:* 1322–1325 (1983).

46 Kabat, E.A.; Wu, T.T.; Reid-Miller, M.; et al.: Sequences of proteins of immunological interest (US Department of Health & Human Services, Washington 1987).

47 Chen, P.P.; Robbins, D.L.; Jirik, F.R.; et al.: Isolation and characterization of a light chain variable region gene for human rheumatoid factors. J. exp. Med. *166:* 1900–1905 (1987).

48 Liu, M.-F.; Robbins, D.L.; Crowley, J.J.; et al.: Characterization of four homologous light chain variable region genes which are related to 6B6.6 idiotype positive human rheumatoid factor light chains. J. Immun. *142:* 688–694 (1989).

49 Schroeder, H.W., Hr.; Hillson, J.L.; Perlmutter, R.M.: Early restriction of the human antibody repertoire. Science *238:* 791–793 (1987).

50 Takahashi, N.; Noma, T.; Honjo, T.: Rearranged immunoglobulin heavy chain variable region (Vh) pseudogene that deletes the second complementarity-determining region. Proc. natn. Acad. Sci. USA *81:* 5194–5198 (1984).

51 Kodaira, M.; Kinashi, T.; Umemura, I.; et al.: Organization and evolution of variable region genes of the human immunoglobulin heavy chain. J. molec. Biol. *190:* 529–541 (1986).

52 Berman, J.E.; Mellis, S.J.; Pollock, R.; et al.: Content and organization of the human Ig VH locus. Definition of three new VH families and linkage to the Ig CH locus. Eur. molec. biol. Org. J. *7:* 727–738 (1988).

53 Chen, P.P.; Liu, M.-F.; Glass, C.A.; et al.: Characterization of two Ig Vh genes which are homologous to human rheumatoid factors. Arthritis Rheum. *32:* 72–76 (1989).

54 Ravetch, J.V.; Siebenlist, U.; Korsmeyer, S.; et al.: Structure of the human immunoglobulin mu locus. Characterization of embryonic and rearranged J and D genes. Cell *27:* 583–591 (1981).

55 Crews, S.; Griffin, J.; Huang, H.; et al.: A single Vh gene segment encodes the immune response to phosphorylcholine. Somatic mutation is correlated with the class of the antibody. Cell *25:* 59–66 (1981).

56 Perlmutter, R.M.; Crews, S.T.; Klotz, J.; et al.: Molecular genetics of anti-carbohydrate antibodies. Ann. Immunol., Paris *135C:* 83–88 (1984).

57 Gearhart, P.J.: The adaptable somatic repertoire. Ann. Immunol., Paris *135C:* 137–142 (1984).

58 Oudin, J.; Cazenave, P.A.: Similar idiotypic specificities in immunoglobulin factions with different antibody functions or even without detectable antibody function. Proc. natn. Acad. Sci. USA *68:* 2616 (1971).

59 Bona, C.A.: Parallel sets and the internal image of antigen within the idiotypic network. Fed. Proc. *43:* 2558–2562 (1984).

60 Agnello, V.; Goni, F.; Barnes, J.L.; et al.: Human rheumatoid factor crossidiotypes. II. Primary structure-dependent crossreactive idiotype, PSL2-CRI, present on Wa monoclonal rheumatoid factors is present on Bla and other IgMk monoclonal autoantibodies. J. exp. Med. *165:* 263–267 (1987).

61 Newkirk, M.M.; Gram, H.; Heinrich, G.F; et al.: The complete protein sequences of the variable regions of the cloned heavy and light chains of a human anti-cytomegalovirus antibody reveal a striking similarity to human rheumatoid factors of the Wa idiotypic family. J. clin. Inves. *81:* 1511 (1988).

62 Kipps, T.J.; Fong, S.; Tomhave, E.; et al.: High frequency expression of a conserved kappa variable region gene in chronic lymphocytic leukemia. Proc. natn. Acad. Sci. USA *84:* 2916–2920 (1987).

63 Kipps, T.J.; Tomhave, E.; Chen, P.P.; et al.: Autoantibody-associated kappa light chain variable region gene expressed in chronic lymphocytic leukemia with little or no somatic mutation. Implications for etiology and immunotherapy. J. exp. Med. *167:* 840–852 (1988).

64 Fong, S.; Gilbertson, T.A.; Hueniken, R.J.; et al.: IgM rheumatoid factor autoantibody and immunoglobulin producing precursor cells in the bone marrow of humans. Cell. Immunol. *95:* 157–172 (1985).

65   Portnoi, D.; Freitas, A.; Holmberg, D.; et al.: Immunocompetent autoreactive B lymphocytes are activated cycling cells in normal mice. J. exp. Med. *164:* 25–35 (1986).
66   Holmberg, D.; Freitas, A.A.; Portnoi, D.; et al.: Antibody repertories of normal BABL/c mice. B lymphocyte populations defined by state of activation. Immunol. Rev. *93:* 147–169 (1986).
67   Shlomchik, M.; Nemazee, D.; Van Snick, J.; et al.: Variable region sequences of murine IgM anti-IgG monoclonal autoantibodies (rheumatoid factors). II. Comparison of hybridomas derived by lipopolysaccharide stimulation and secondary protein immunization. J. exp. Med. *165:* 970–987 (1987).
68   Painter, C.; Monestier, M.; Bonin, B.; et al.: Functional and molecular studies of V genes expressed in autoantibodies. Immunol. Rev. *94:* 75–98 (1986).
69   Manser, T.; Wysocki, L.J.; Gidley, T.; et al.: The molecular evolution of the immune response. Immunol. Today *6:* 94–101 (1985).
70   Tzioufas, A.G.; Manoussakis, M.N.; Costello, R.; et al.: Cryoglobulinemia in autoimmune rheumatic diseases. Arthritis Rheum. *29:* 1098 (1986).
71   Talal, N.; Bunim, J.: The development of malignant lymphoma in Sjogren's syndrome. Am. J. Med. *36:* 529–540 (1964).

Pojen P. Chen, PhD, Departments of Basic and Clinical Research, Scripps Clinic and Research Foundation, 10666 North Torrey Pines Road, La Jolla, CA 92037 (USA)

Carson DA, Chen PP, Kipps TJ (eds): Idiotypes in Biology and Medicine.
Chem Immunol. Basel, Karger, 1990, vol 48, pp 82–108

Idiotypes in Systemic Lupus Erythematosus

Clues for Understanding Etiology and Pathogenicity

*R. Shefner, A. Manheimer-Lory, A. Davidson, E. Paul, C. Aranow,
J. Katz, B. Diamond*

Albert Einstein College of Medicine, Bronx, N.Y., USA

Introduction

For many years antibody molecules were characterized by their antigenic
specificity. Then pioneering work by Kunkel and Oudin demonstrated that
antigenic determinants exist within the variable region [1–4]. These determinants are called idiotypes and can be used to construct a profile of an
antibody molecule. An antibody molecule can, therefore, be characterized
not only by its antigenic specificity but also by its idiotype. In general,
idiotypic determinants are recognized by both B cells and T cells and
constitute a target for regulation within the immune system [5–7]. An
idiotypic analysis of immunoglobulin molecules can be particularly fruitful
since one can simultaneously learn about the structure, function, molecular
genetics, and regulation of antibodies of a defined antigenic specificity.

Generation of Antibody Diversity and the Ontogeny of a B Cell Response

The immunoglobulin heavy chain variable gene locus on chromosome
12 in mouse and chromosome 14 in man is composed of 3 noncontiguous
sets of genetic elements [8–10]. The variable region (V), diversity (D), and
joining (J) segments are separated from each other by many kilobases of
DNA. During B cell development, members of these three gene clusters
undergo an ordered DNA rearrangement to form a VDJ gene sequence that
encodes the intact heavy chain variable region [11–13]. In the mouse, where

immunoglobulin genes have been most extensively studied, it has been estimated that there exist between 200 and 1,000 V_H genes, approximately 12–20 D_H segments and 4 functional J_H genes [14–17]. The immunoglobulin light chain variable region genes located on chromosomes 6 (k) and 16 (λ) in mouse, and chromosomes 2 (k) and chromosome 22 (λ) in man, have only 2 sets of genetic elements V and J [18–22]. These genes also undergo DNA rearrangement to form a light chain variable region. The vast majority of murine antibodies possess a kappa-light chain. There are approximately 200 V_K genes in mouse and 4 functional J_k genes [16, 23, 24].

Diversification of antibody molecules generates an antibody repertoire protective against an apparently infinite range of invading foreign antigens. Antibody diversity is generated by several mechanisms: (1) random association of heavy and light chains; (2) utilization of different V, D and J segments to form each heavy chain variable region and different V and J segments to form each light chain variable region, and (3) alternative splice sites at the junction between the V, and D, and J segments in the heavy chain and between the V and J segments in the light chain. Alt and Baltimore described the addition of nontemplate derived nucleotides at the V-D and D-J junctions of heavy chain variable regions. Addition of nucleotides can also occur at the V_K-J_K junction. These nucleotides (N sequences) are added by terminal deoxytransferase during DNA rearrangement [25–27].

Gene conversion, gene replacement, and somatic point mutation are three additional mechanisms which expand the immune repertoire [28–41, 50, 51]. Gene conversion describes a microcombination process in which a discrete part of one gene is incorporated into another gene through a nonreciprocal exchange event, thereby altering the sequence within one of the genes. This process is responsible for diversification of the chicken λ-light chain repertoire where a large number of pseudogenes provide donor sequences for one funtional Vλ gene [31, 35, 36]. While there are few indications that gene conversion contributes greatly to the diversity of the murine antibody response [34, 42, 43], it may be an important mechanism of diversification in man as an apparently large number of V_H pseudogenes exist within the human V_H gene locus [44, 45]. Gene replacement is a related process in which all or part of a novel V gene replaces the V of an already rearranged VDJ or VJ [32, 33]. The importance of this process in vivo is not known. Finally, somatic point mutation of VDJ or VJ sequences is a major mechanism of diversification and in the mouse has been estimated to occur at a frequency of 10^{-3} base pairs/cell/generation [29, 37–41]. As these mechanisms may all result in amino acid substitutions within the variable region, they can have profound effects on the antigenic and idiotypic specificity of the antibody gene product [46, 47].

Each mechanism for generating diversity is characteristic of a particular stage in B cell development. Combinatorial and junctional mechanisms generate diversity in the B cell repertoire prior to antigen exposure. B cells encountering antigen during a primary immune response generally produce antibodies encoded by germline gene sequences without somatic diversification [48]. Only after a B cell is exposed to antigen does somatic point mutation come into play [29, 38, 39, 41, 49–51]. The primary immune response consists, in general, of low affinity and polyspecific IgM antibodies. The maturation of antibody response is characterized by the development of higher affinity and more monospecific IgG antibodies [52–55].

It is thought that somatic mutation occurs as IgM antibodies undergo a heavy chain class switch event to become IgG antibodies. While there is not an absolute requirement for isotype switching to accompany somatic mutation, IgG antibodies display somatic mutations more often than IgM antibodies [29, 38, 39, 49, 50, 56, 57]. They are of higher affinity and more monospecific than the parental IgM antibodies, because antigen selectively expands those B cells producing the highest affinity antibodies [39, 51]. Studies of hybridomas generated from mice immunized with the hapten 2-phenyloxazalone, for example, show that somatically mutated antibodies are rare 7 days after immunization but are found with high frequency in the late primary and in the secondary response [39]. The highly mutated antibodies demonstrated a higher affinity for hapten than the germline-encoded precursors. Somatic mutations are generally clustered in the 3 hypervariable or complementarity-determining regions (CDRs), areas that are presumed to be in contact with antigen [59, 60]. Framework regions which do not contact antigen accumulate fewer mutations.

It is possible to analyze the mutations within the variable region of an antibody gene and speculate on the forces acting upon the B cell. If somatic mutations of immunoglobulin variable region genes were random, the ratio of mutations in the CDRs that alter the amino acid (replacement mutations) to mutations that do not alter the amino acid (silent mutations) would be approximately 3 to 1. Activation of B cells by mitogens or polyclonal B cell activators, will lead to a replacement to silent mutation ratio of 3 to 1 [61]. If the B cell response is activated by specific antigen, that antigen will select for those muations that create a high-affinity antibody, presumably by preferentially stimulating proliferation of those B cell clones that make the higher affinity antibodies, and display an increased number of replacement mutations [39]. Using this type of analysis it is possible to determine whether an immune response is due to a nonspecific activation of B cells or to an antigen-driven process.

Variable Region Gene Families

Immunoglobulin variable (V) region genes are grouped into families based on their DNA sequence homology; 80% homology is required to place V region genes within the same family. The areas of antigen contact, the CDRs, are the regions that differ most between members of the same family, while the framework regions are highly conserved. In general, antibodies encoded by members of the same V region gene family share many of the same antigenic determinants on their V regions and are therefore idiotypically related and may be coregulated.

In mice 10 heavy chain V region gene families and 20–35 V_k light chain gene families have been identified to date [23, 62]. Variable region families differ dramatically in size. The J558 family consists of 200–1,000 members while the 441-4 family has only two [15, 17]. It is likely, however, that not all variable region genes are used in the functional antibody repertoire. Some members are clearly pseudogenes and may function only as donor sequences in gene conversion events [30, 63]. In mouse it seems that the members of each V_H region family are contiguous [44, 64, 157]. Alt and colleagues [65] and others [66] have suggested that the families are preferentially expressed at different times in the ontogeny of the immune system. Those V_H region gene families located most proximal to the constant region genes appear to be used earliest in the immune response and the more distant 5′ genes are used later in the development of the B cell repertoire.

The organization of the human heavy chain immunoglobulin variable region locus has recently been explored by several laboratories [67, 68] and at least 6 V_H families have been identified. Each family contains a different number of genes: $V_H1(20–25)$, $V_H2(5–10)$, $V_H3(25–30)$, $V_H4(6–10)$, $V_H5(2–3)$, $V_H6(1–2)$. A seventh V_H family may also exist [68]. The organization of V_K light chain genes in man has been studied as well and there appear to be at least 5 V_K families [69–72] which lie in two reduplicated regions and contain at least 50 V_K genes. In humans, it is thought that members of the different V region gene families are interspersed [45, 67]. It is not known if some genes are preferentially utilized in the neonatal repertoire and others later in development.

Autoantibodies in Systemic Lupus Erythematosus

Systemic lupus erythematosus (SLE), has been considered the prototype of an autoimmune disease and thus much of the data on autoantibodies has been derived from investigations of human lupus and murine models of the disease. A wide spectrum of autoantibodies is present in SLE. Antibodies to various cells (erythrocytes, platelets, lymphocytes, neurons, hepatocytes) and to cytoplasmic constituents (cytoskeletal elements, mitochondria, microsomes), have been identified in patients with SLE [73, 74, 86, 87, 89]. The most prominent subset of SLE autoantibodies, however, are antinuclear antibodies including anti-Sm, anti-RNP, anti-cardiolipin, anti-RO/SSA, anti-La/SSB and anti-DNA/RNA [76–89, 121, 149–151]. Many studies have attempted to elucidate the molecular and cellular mechanisms involved in generating these autoantibodies, and the role each specificity plays (if any) in the pathogenesis of the autoimmune disease.

Anti-Sm antibodies are a specific marker for SLE although only 1/3 of patients make antibodies with this specificity [75]. The Sm antigen, a complex consisting of small nuclear RNA and protein molecules (termed 'snRNP'), has been isolated and purified from nuclear extracts by affinity chromatography [76–78]. The antigenic determinants on Sm reside in the protein portion and are recognized by both human and murine anti-Sm antibodies. Anti-RNP, a closely related antibody directed against another snRNP, is also frequently found in SLE patients [79]. Titers of these antibodies do not correlate well with patterns of disease activity and it is still unresolved what role, if any, these antibodies play in pathogenesis.

Anti-Ro/SSA and anti-La/SSB antibodies comprise another family of antinuclear antibodies [80, 81]. Ro/SSA is also a ribonuclear protein complex [80]. Antigenicity has again been attributed to the protein portion of the complex. Anti-Ro antibodies are often found in patients with Sjogrens syndrome and in a subset of SLE patients with predominantly cutaneous disease. Anti-Ro antibodies have been strongly implicated in the development of congenital heart block in infants whose mothers possess this antibody.

The most common autoantibody in SLE is antibody to double-stranded (ds) DNA. Reactivity to native or dsDNA is generally considered a diagnostic marker for lupus since anti-dsDNA antibodies rarely occur in other clinical conditions [75]. Anti-DNA antibodies are thought to be pathogenic as anti-dsDNA antibodies are deposited in the skin and kidneys of SLE patients and titers increase and decrease during disease flares and remissions, respectively [84]. While antibodies specific for dsDNA are pathogenic, they are often found in conjunction with anti-denatured or single-stranded (ss) DNA antibodies, polynucleotide specific antibodies, as well as antibodies specific to an alternative DNA conformation, Z-DNA [82]. The nature of the antigenic epitopes on DNA is still not clear. Some studies suggest that the bases contribute to the fine specificity of the antibodies [85]. Alternatively, Stollar et al. [83] have suggested that the phosphate backbone is the structurally significant target of anti-dsDNA antibodies, thus accounting for the wide cross-reactivity of monoclonal anti-DNA antibodies with molecules containing a phosphorylated epitope. One of the most puzzling features of this system is the lack of immunogenicity of DNA itself. Immunization of mice with DNA does not elicit the anti-dsDNA antibodies typically found in SLE. Immunization of mice with cardiolipin has, however, been shown to result in production of anti-dsDNA antibodies thereby providing evidence for the hypothesis that phosphate epitopes are the antigenic determinants on DNA, and presenting a model in which a non-DNA antigen can lead to production of anti-DNA antibodies [88]. Many anti-dsDNA antibodies present in SLE serum, however, do not cross-react with cardiolipin, so there must be additional antigenic epitopes on DNA. It is hoped that further studies on the fine specificity of anti-DNA antibodies may help elucidate the antigen(s) responsible for eliciting their production.

For many years SLE was thought to be a disease of abnormal polyclonal B cell activation because individuals with SLE produce such a wide variety of autoantibodies. As murine models of SLE became available (the MRL/1pr, NZB/NZW F_1 and BXSB mice), an alternative hypothesis for autoreactivity arose. It was proposed that SLE might be a disease of regulatory T cells [90, 91, 153]. Data from in vivo experiments using a variety of methods to deplete autoimmune mice of T cells suggested that the production of autoantibodies in at least some strains of mice [91–94] was markedly enhanced by T lymphocytes. Similarly, in vitro experiments analyzing autoantibody production by B cells alone and by B cells cocultured with T cells suggested T cell participation in the autoantibody response [95, 96]. Other studies in mice indicated that B cell hyperactivity is prominent and ascribed a more limited role to T cells in the abnormal immune response [97, 98]. It has, therefore, remained a matter of controversy whether the B cells in SLE are stimulated to produce autoantibodies by T cells and by antigen or whether they are nonspecifically activated. Moreover, if antigen is necessary for the development of autoimmunity, it remains unknown whether the antigen is an autoantigen or a foreign antigen [99–101]. Studies adddressing these questions will help define the relationship of autoantibodies present in an immunologic disease to normal protective antibodies.

Natural Autoantibodies

While autoantibodies can easily be detected in the serum of patients with SLE, recent studies have shown that even normal individuals have B cells capable of expressing autoantibodies. A number of laboratories have used peripheral blood or tonsillar B cells of normal individuals to generate human B cell hybridomas or Epstein-Barr virus (EBV)-transformed B cell lines producing antibodies which bind to the nuclear autoantigens that define SLE antibodies [102–105]. Interestingly, these 'natural' autoantibodies, so called because they arise in normal nonautoimmune individuals, can share idiotypic determinants with the autoantibodies of similar specificity present in SLE serum [106]. While idiotypically similar, they nevertheless differ from SLE autoantibodies in a variety of ways that suggest that natural autoantibodies form part of the preimmune repertoire and that the autoantibodies of autoimmune disease are antibodies made by B cells following exposure to antigen [105, 107]. Natural autoantibodies are almost exclusively IgM, while SLE autoantibodies are primarily IgG [84, 104, 108, 109–111]. Natural autoantibodies have much lower affinity for antigen than the antibodies of autoimmune disease [84, 111]. Furthermore, natural autoantibodies are polyspecific; they bind to a number of autoantigens [87–89, 105, 111–113]. Natural anti-DNA antibodies, for example, will bind to double-stranded DNA, single-stranded DNA, cardiolipin, and cytoskeletal proteins such as vimentin, while the pathogenic autoantibodies of autoimmune disease tend to be more monospecific. Natural autoantibodies appear to be encoded by germline gene sequences [107]; the nature of the differences between natural autoantibodies and autoantibodies in disease leads one to suspect that the autoantibodies in disease are encoded by somatically mutated genes [58, 114]. It is intriguing to speculate that natural autoantibodies are, in fact, the precursors of the autoantibodies in disease [115].

Idiotypic Analyses of Anti-DNA Antibodies

In recent years hybridoma technology has been employed to generate B cell lines making monoclonal autoantibodies and lines making anti-idiotypes to autoantibodies. These reagents have been used to study the relationship between antibodies directed to foreign antigen and directed to self antigen in murine and human SLE and so to begin to understand the etiology of SLE.

Idiotypic analysis permits one to identify variable region determinants commonly expressed on antibodies in disease states, to analyze the structure of such antibodies, to obtain clues about their genetic origins, and to dissect the relationship of particular antibody subsets to pathogenesis [58, 114, 116–151]. Anti-idiotypes were first used in studies of SLE to examine anti-DNA antibodies in murine models of lupus. Schwartz and colleagues demonstrated restricted idiotypy on anti-DNA antibodies produced by B cell hybridomas from MRL/1pr mice [138, 139]. The idiotypes that characterized anti-DNA antibodies were also present on antibodies without specificity for DNA and even on antibodies present in the serum of nonautoimmune mice [140]. A number of other laboratories have identified cross-reactive idiotypes on anti-DNA antibodies from MRL/1pr or NZB/W F_1 mice [123, 141–145]. In most cases, it appears that idiotypes present on anti-DNA antibodies are present on non-DNA-binding antibodies present in the autoimmune mice and on antibodies in nonautoimmune strains of mice [140, 145].

Idiotypic studies in human SLE also demonstrated the detection of 'public' or cross-reactive idiotypic determinants on anti-DNA antibodies [58]. Studies from our own laboratory have identified three dominant idiotypes which are present on anti-DNA antibodies from unrelated lupus patients and are present also at high frequency on myeloma proteins. By isolating anti-DNA antibodies from the plasma of patients with SLE and using these antibodies to immunize mice, it was possible to exploit standard hybridoma technology to produce monoclonal anti-idiotypes to anti-dsDNA antibodies. The first anti-idiotype produced by this means was the 3I antibody which recognizes a determinant on kappa-light chains on anti-DNA antibodies in SLE. The 3I anti-idiotype detects elevated titers of 3I-reactive antibodies in 80% of SLE sera with anti-DNA activity [58]. In these sera a large percent of the anti-DNA antibodies bear the 3I idiotype; however, 50% of 3I reactive antibodies do not bind DNA. There is, therefore, an idiotypic relationship between anti-DNA antibodies and antibodies with other antigenic specificities. Elevated titers of 3I reactivity are also present in clinically unaffected family members in SLE kindreds [146]. These idiotypic antibodies, in general, are not DNA binding and must be presumed to form part of a repertoire of antibodies to foreign antigen.

The F4 anti-idiotype recognizes a determinant on the heavy chain of most 3I-reactive cationic anti-DNA antibodies and shows high titered reactivity with 60% of SLE sera [114]. 3I-reactive, F4-reactive antibodies are more likely to bind DNA and to be cationic than 3I-reactive, F4-nonreactive antibodies. Ebling and Hahn [147] have suggested that cationic anti-DNA antibodies are preferentially deposited in the kidney and are therefore more pathogenic. 3I-reactive, F4-reactive anti-DNA antibodies may be more pathogenic than 3I-reactive anti-DNA antibodies that lack the F4 idiotype.

The 8.12 anti-idiotype recognizes a determinant on lambda-light chains and thus identifies a different subset of anti-DNA antibodies [128]. 8.12 reactivity, elevated in 50% of SLE sera, is also preferentially found on cationic anti-DNA antibodies. Approximately 50% of 8.12-reactive antibodies in SLE sera have no specificity for DNA, again suggesting an idiotypic relationship between antibodies of different specificities.

Schwartz and colleagues generated human B cell hybridomas from peripheral blood lymphocytes of individuals with SLE. One line, 16/6, made a DNA-binding antibody which was used to generate both polyclonal rabbit anti-idiotypic serum and a murine monoclonal anti-idiotype. Using these anti-idiotypic reagents, one can detect elevated titers of antibodies bearing the 16/6 idiotype in unrelated patients with SLE [116]. Isenberg et al. [137] showed that clinically unaffected individuals in SLE kindreds also have elevated titers of the 16/6 idiotype. In these family members lacking anti-DNA activity, the 16/6 idiotypic antibodies presumably form part of a normal antibody repertoire. While the antigenic specificity of these antibodies in normal serum is not known, Naparstek et al. [130] showed that an IgM macroglobulin, WEA, that binds to a polysaccharide antigen on the Klebsiella bacterium cell wall also bears the 16/6 idiotype. Furthermore, El-Roiey et al. [148] demonstrated that individuals with Klebsiella infections have antibodies of the 16/6 idiotype and antibodies with affinity for denatured DNA. Bell et al. [127], using a human monoclonal anti-DNA antibody, produced an anti-idiotypic reagent which recognizes determinants present on anti-DNA antibodies in 85% of SLE patients and also on non-DNA-binding antibodies in serum of their first-degree relatives. Rauch et al. [117] identified a public idiotype which is present both on anti-DNA antibodies and rheumatoid factor and may be a marker for more than one autoimmune disease. Yet another idiotype has been identified on both anti-DNA and anti-Sm antibodies [129].

These studies lead to several conclusions. First, anti-DNA antibodies possess public or cross-reactive idiotypes. While this was not particularly surprising in studies of inbred strains of mice, it was in no way predictable that unrelated members of an outbred human population would make highly structurally homologous antibodies to any self antigen. Despite differences in both the MHC molecules of these unrelated individuals, and in their T cell repertoires, the antibodies directed to DNA or Sm or Ro are structurally similar. It has become apparent that antibodies of any given specificity will bear cross-reactive idiotypes in unrelated individuals; this idiotypic related-ness of antibodies of a defined specificity was first observed in studies of autoantibodies. Since antibodies that share idiotypic determinants are gener-ally encoded by highly homologous variable region genes, the idiotypic relatedness of autoantibodies means not only a structural similarity at the protein level but, in all probability, a genetic relationship as well [6].

Secondly, it is clear from the studies described that a population of idiotypically related antibodies contains antibodies of more than one anti-genic specificity. One implication of this observation is that the same or highly homologous variable region genes are used to make autoantibodies and antibodies to non-self antigens and that there are probably no 'autoanti-body genes', genes used exclusively for the production of autoantibodies [152, 154, 155]. Further there may be no antibody genes specific to autoim-mune kindreds. Idiotypic antibodies without autoantibody specificity are present at unusually high titer in the family members of lupus patients. The interpretation of this observation is complicated by the fact that high-titered expression of idiotype can be found not only in first-degree relatives but also occasionally in a spouse [146]. While there appears, therefore, to be a genetic determination of variable region gene usage, other factors also play a role in selection of an antibody repertoire. Finally, idiotypic studies suggest a relationship between antibodies to DNA and antibodies to infectious patho-gens. Furthermore, they suggest a possible etiologic role for infectious agents in triggering autoantibody production [99–101, 156].

The Molecular Genetic Origins of Autoantibodies

It has been proposed by Jerne [115] that the immunoglobulin germline gene repertoire is anti-self and that mutations of these anti-self antibodies are required to generate the repertoire of antibodies to foreign antigens. Alterna-tively, it has also been proposed that anti-self specificity is generated by somatic mutation of germline genes [154].

Even if there are no genes that encode only autoantibodies, it appears from some studies that certain genes or gene families are preferentially used to encode autoantibodies. By analyzing rheumatoid factor-secreting hybridomas from MRL/1pr mice, Arant et al. [158] showed restricted V_H gene usage in 6 of 9 hybridomas. These hybridomas derived their heavy chain variable region from members of the 36-60 V_H gene family, a family used in A/J mice, to make antibodies that react with the hapten azophenylarsonate. However, in a similar study Aguado et al. [159] examined the antigenic specificity and V_H gene usage of rheumatoid factors and found that the J558 V_H gene family was used by 32 of 35 rheumatoid factor-secreting hybridomas derived from three different mouse strains. Because this family is the largest in the mouse V_H repertoire and is said to encode more than 60% of all mouse immunoglobulins, the significance of this apparent genetic restriction is unclear. Monestier et al. [160] analyzed a panel of 61 autoantibodies of various specificities from different mouse strains for expression of a shared cross-reactive idiotype, IdX. They found a preferential usage of the J558 family, the QPC52 family, and the 7183 family. The latter two families are located at the J_H proximal end of the heavy chain variable gene locus. It is interesting to note that the 7183 family is used infrequently by mature B cells but frequently by B cells early in development. The authors interpret these findings to indicate that autoantibodies may preferentially arise from a population of immature B cells.

In our own laboratory we are presently characterizing antibodies both DNA binding and non-DNA binding human antibodies expressing one or two dominant SLE idiotypes, 3I (V_K associated), or F4 (V_H associated) derived by EBV transformation of cells from lupus patients and patients with myeloma whose myeloma protein bears an autoantibody-associated idiotype. Preliminary results do not indicate preferential usage of one V_H gene family to encode antibodies in these EBV-transformed lines. Analysis of the V_k genes utilized, however, indicates that most but not all 3I reactive lines use a member of the $V_K 1$ family. Because $V_K 1$ genes are used by idiotypic non-DNA-binding antibodies, it is likely that in humans, as in mice, V genes used by anti-DNA antibodies are not solely utilized to produce autoantibodies [manuscript in preparation].

Support for the theory that autoreactivity is encoded within the germline and that mutation is directed away from autoreactivity in the anti-DNA system comes primarily from data derived from nonautoimmune strains of mice. Schwartz and Gefter and their colleagues studied B cells expressing a V_H gene that encodes a dominant cross-reactive idiotype (CRI) in the anti-arsonate response in A/J mice [107]. They analyzed hybridomas from mitogen-stimulated B cells from A/J mice that produce antibodies that use the V_H gene which encodes the CRI. Approximately one-half of the CRI V_H hybridoma studied bound single-stranded DNA, while none bound arsonate. Molecular analysis of the V_H genes in these B cells showed them to be unmutated. When hybridomas were derived from mice immunized with arsonate, the B cells expressing the CRI V_H produced arosonate-binding antibodies which showed little or no cross-reactivity with DNA and which all possessed somatically mutated VDJ variable region genes. The authors interpret this observation to mean that anti-DNA specificity resides within the germline and that mutation leads to loss of autoreactivity. Alternatively, a more conservative interpretation might be that antibodies to DNA can be encoded by a germline V_H gene, and that mutations increasing the affinity of the antibody encoded by this V_H gene for arsonate concomitantly decrease its binding to DNA. It is possible that other mutations which do not lead to the production of arsonate-binding antibodies do indeed lead to antibodies with higher affinity for DNA, and that high-affinity DNA binding may be somatically generated. Studies of neonatal mice have also provided data suggesting a germline origin for autoantibodies [161]. B cell hybridomas from neonatal mice are thought to represent the antibody repertoire of the animal prior to exposure to antigen and prior to somatic mutation of antibody genes. The B cells from neonatal animals produce IgM antibodies many of which show low-affinity reactivity with a number of autoantigens. The antibodies are not pathogenic themselves and it remains unclear how they relate to the pathogenic antibodies of autoimmune disease.

Diamond and Scharff [46] have suggested that autoantibodies may arise by somatic mutation of antibodies to non-self antigens. They observed in vitro that a somatic mutation in the S107 anti-phosphorylcholine (PC) antibody leads to a loss of binding to PC and to the acquisition of binding to dsDNA. A single nucleotide change resulting in a single amino acid substitution of glutamic acid to alanine in position 35 of the first CDR is responsible for the change in antigenic specificity. This was the first observation to suggest that somatic mutation might be a mechanism for generating autoreactivity. Shlomchik et al. [162, 163] subsequently examined the variable regions of rheumatoid factors from MRL/lpr mice and found them to reflect the accumulation of somatic mutations. In fact, it appears that the mutations in these antibodies have been selected by antigen as the ratio of replacement to silent mutations is greater than that expected from random mutation. Similarly, Shlomchik et al. studied anti-DNA antibodies produced by spleen cell hybridomas from MRL/lpr mice and found these also to be encoded by mutated variable region genes, and to have a replacement to silent mutation ratio of approximately seven to one [164]. While this observation again suggests that autoantibodies are antigen selected, it is not necessary that DNA be the selecting antigen. It may be that mutated antibodies are elicited by foreign antigen and yet cross-react with DNA.

Behar and Scharff [165], studying anti-DNA antibodies from NZB/NZW F_1 mice, also demonstrated that the antibodies possess somatic mutations. They immunized NZB/NZW F_1 mice with PC which elicits antibodies using a V_H gene from the T15 gene family and, after cloning and sequencing the germline genes of the T15 V_H gene family, were able to show unequivocally that anti-DNA hybridoma antibodies encoded by T15 V_H genes show the accumulation of somatic mutations. They also found a replacement to silent mutation ratio that suggests a role for antigen selection. Studies of anti-Sm antibodies in murine SLE have led to similar conclusions. The anti-Sm response in MRL/lpr mice seems to be almost exclusively an IgG response and there appear to be no IgM precursor cells with specificity for Sm [166]. The acquisition of Sm binding apparently coincides with the switch from IgM to IgG, an event associated with the accumulation of somatic mutations.

Studies of human autoantibodies have also addressed the question of the molecular genetics of autoantibody formation and the interpretations of the data are conflicting. The 16/6 human anti-DNA antibody has been investigated on a molecular level; its V_H gene sequence is 99% homologous to a previously sequenced germline V_HIII gene, V_H26 [134]. One additional 16/6 idiotypic antibody also appears to be encoded by an unmutated gene [152]. Studies of human rheumatoid factors also provide evidence for germline gene utilization by autoantibodies [135]. A high percentage of light chains from monoclonal rheumatoid factors made by patients with B cell malignancies is encoded by a small number of conserved germline genes. However, when one examines rheumatoid factor light chains present in patients with rheumatoid arthritis, a wider variety of V_K gene families is utilized and the antibodies no longer appear to have absolute fidelity to germline genes.

In our laboratory, studies of 3I idiotypic antibodies have suggested that somatic mutation plays a role in the production of DNA-binding antibodies. When we examined 3I-reactive myeloma proteins, we found that a significantly greater percentage of IgG 3I-reactive antibodies bound DNA than did IgM 3I-reactive antibodies. Furthermore, there is a marked increase in the charge heterogeneity of the 3I-reactive kappa-light chains of IgG antibodies compared to the 3I-reactive kappa-light chains of IgM antibodies [58]. We believe that somatic mutation is the mechanism underlying the increased heterogeneity of idiotypic light chains on IgG antibodies and is also responsible for the acquisition of DNA binding by the IgG antibodies. Nucleic acid sequence analysis of a 3I- and F4-reactive anti-DNA antibody reveals it to have extensively mutated from the most homologous reported germline genes. It is important to remember, however, that although several human autoantibody gene sequences have been published, the appropriate germline genes have not yet been obtained from individuals with autoimmune disease. This precludes one from knowing the degree of polymorphism of homologous germline genes and whether certain polymorphisms are present in autoimmune kindreds and predispose to autoimmunity. The sequence analysis of the 3I- and F4-reactive anti-DNA antibody further reveals a replacement to silent mutation ratio of 2:1 in the framework regions and 9:0 in the heavy chains CDRs and 15:3 in the light chain CDRs. This suggests an antigen-selected antibody. It is clear that sequence data of many autoantibodies in conjunction with germline sequences will be necessary to establish the relative contribution of somatic mutation to the generation of high-affinity anti-DNA antibodies and to the formation of pathogenic antibodies.

Anti-Idiotypes in Diagnosis

Since antibodies bearing autoantibody-associated idiotypes need not have autoantigen specificity and may be present in high titers in normal individuals, can anti-idiotypes help in the diagnosis or management of individuals with SLE? Our laboratory studied 13 patients at two times in their disease, once when anti-DNA activity was present and once when no anti-DNA antibodies were detectable using conventional antigen-binding assays [121]. All 13 patients showed elevated titers of 3I reactivity when anti-DNA antibodies were present; 6 patients had normal titers when anti-DNA activity was no longer present. Seven patients retained elevated titers of 3I reactivity even when no anti-DNA binding was detected with conventional assays. By examining the sera under conditions that dissociate immune complexes, it was possible to show in all sera with elevated titers of 3I-reactive antibodies that there were anti-DNA antibodies present. This study suggests that assays for expression of particular idiotypes may be an important adjunct to antigen-binding assays in analyzing SLE sera; if anti-idiotypes do not bind to the antigen-binding site of the antibody, they may detect antibodies present in immune complexes which would not be found in antigen-binding assays.

Studies in the 16/6 system have shown that one can monitor relapses and remissions in disease activity with an idiotypic analysis of serum [116]. These data suggest that despite the fact that anti-idiotypes may recognize nonautoantibodies as well as autoantibodies, they may be useful in monitoring disease activity and response to therapy.

It is also possible that one might use anti-idiotypes to identify determinants on anti-DNA antibodies that are not present on antibodies in a normal immune response or to characterize a pathogenic subset of anti-DNA antibodies. Ebling and Hahn [147] have clearly shown in murine lupus that anti-idiotypes can distinguish between anti-DNA antibodies that deposit in the glomerulus and anti-DNA antibodies that do not. The human PR4 idiotype which characterizes an anti-ssDNA antibody derived from a patient with leprosy, is elevated in SLE sera and in sera from individuals with other autoimmune diseases [132]. The PR4 idiotype is not elevated in unaffected family members in SLE kindreds. It appears that this idiotype identifies autoantibodies and may identify pathogenic antibodies. Likewise, the F4 and 8.12 anti-idiotypes studied in our laboratory recognize cationic antibodies. While they recognize some antibodies without DNA specificity, the anti-DNA antibodies they bind may be pathogenic. Further studies are necessary to determine the relationship of these idiotypic determinants to pathogenicity. Anti-idiotypes have an as yet untapped potential as diagnostic reagents. The next several years will no doubt see studies designed to define this potential.

Idiotypic Regulation of Anti-DNA Antibodies

The network hypothesis, described 20 years ago by Jerne [167], suggests that antibody idiotypes are targets for immune regulation by both B and T cells. Several investigators have demonstrated a genetic basis for the idiotype network [168, 169]. Using GAT as antigen, Schiff et al. [168] found that immunization either with antigen or with anti-idiotype (Ab2) led to the generation of hybridomas expressing the same germline genes. Similarly, Margolies et al. [169] showed that immunization with either the hapten *p*-azophenyl arsonate or an anti-idiotype to arsonate-binding antibodies elicits antibodies sharing with each other 95% DNA sequence homology.

Immunization with anti-idiotype can, in fact, either suppress a response to a particular antigen or augment the response, depending on the dose of anti-idiotype. High doses of a monoclonal anti-idiotypic antibody suppress the production of idiotypic antibody in mice whereas low doses lead to higher antibody titers [170]. The fact that anti-idiotypic antibody can lead to a reduction in expression of idiotypic antibody presents a potential approach to specific immunologic intervention in SLE. Hahn and Ebling [141] injected NZB/NZW F_1 mice with anti-idiotype to anti-DNA antibodies. Treatment with anti-idiotype did indeed cause a temporary reduction in expression of anti-DNA antibodies. Eventually, despite a continued reduction in expression of idiotypic antibodies, the expression of anti-DNA antibodies rose to titers seen in untreated mice and glomerulonephritis progressed.

Schoenfeld and Mozes recently reported that a human anti-DNA antibody when injected into a nonautoimmune mouse can cause production of murine idiotypic anti-DNA antibodies and autoimmune disease [171]. Presumably, the anti-DNA antibody elicited anti-idiotype which in turn elicited murine idiotypic antibodies. The importance of this observation is twofold. First it demonstrates that autoantibodies can be regulated by anti-idiotypes in a fashion similar to antibodies to foreign antigen. Second, it suggests that anti-DNA antibodies may be produced in an idiotype network rather than arising in response to either DNA itself or some cross-reactive antigen.

Our laboratory has shown that incubation of peripheral blood lymphocytes in vitro with a monoclonal anti-idiotype, 3I, directed to anti-DNA antibodies will decrease production of anti-DNA antibodies. It is not yet clear if the anti-idiotype acts on the B cell or the T cell but the data provide strong support for the potential of anti-idiotypes in regulation.

Relationship between Autoantibodies and the Immunoglobulins Expressed by Malignant B Cells

It has been reported for many years that individuals with B cell malignancies express an uncommonly high frequency of autoantibodies. Idiotypic analyses of myeloma proteins have also shown a high frequency of autoantibody-associated idiotypes on the myeloma proteins themselves. When we used our 3I anti-idiotypes to anti-DNA antibodies to analyze myeloma proteins [58], we found that approximately 10% of myeloma proteins express each anti-DNA-associated idiotype. This raises a very important but as yet unanswered question. If these idiotypes are present on less than 1% of normal serum immunoglobulin, does their increased expression on myeloma proteins mean that B cells expressing these idiotypes more often undergo malignant transformation or does it mean that B cells expressing these idiotypes are, in general, down-regulated? Unfortunately, precursor frequencies of idiotype bearing B cells have not yet been calculated, and so this question cannot yet be answered.

Conclusion

The study of genetic mechanisms involved in the autoimmune response has been greatly facilitated by monoclonal antibody technology. DNA sequence analysis can now define variable region gene usage in autoantibodies, the structural basis for auto-antigen specificity, as well as the role of somatic mutation in generating autoreactivity. Idiotypic analyses of autoantibodies have not yet yielded information about a possible etiologic agent(s) in SLE but the genetic relatedness of anti-self and anti-foreign antibodies suggests that continued idiotypic analyses may lead to etiologic candidates. Finally, one may yet be able to improve diagnosis with anti-idiotypes and eventually to manipulate the immune system through idiotype regulation.

References

1 Kunkel, H.G.; Mannik, M.; Williams, R.C.: Individual antigenic specificity of isolated antibodies. Science *140:* 1218 (1963).
2 Capra, J.D.; Kehoe, J.M.; Winchester, J.R.; Kunkel, H.G.: Structure-function relationships among anti-gamma globulin antibodies. Ann. N.Y. Acad. Sci. *190:* 371 (1971).
3 Oudin, J.; Michel, M.: Une nouvelle forme d'allotypie des globulines γ du sérum de lapin apparemment liée à la fonction et à la spécificité anticorps. C.r. hebd. Séanc. Acad. Sci., Paris *257:* 805 (1963).
4 Oudin, J.; Cazenave, P.A.: Similar idiotypic specificities in immunoglobulin fractions with different antibody functions or even without detectable antibody function. Proc. natn. Acad. Sci. USA *68:* 2616 (1971).
5 Urbain, J.; Wuilmart, C.: Some thoughts on idiotypic networks and immunoregulation. Immunol. Today *3:* 88 (1982).
6 Rajewsky, K.; Takemori, T.: Genetics, expression and function of idiotypes. A. Rev. Immunol. *1:* 569 (1983).
7 Bottomly, K.: All idiotypes are equal, but some are more equal than others. Immunol. Rev. *79:* 45 (1984).
8 Sakano, H.; Maki, R.; Kurósawa, Y.; Roeder, W.; Tonegawa, S.: Two types of somatic recombination are necessary for the generation of complete immunoglobulin heavy-chain genes. Nature, Lond. *286:* 676 (1980).

9 Early, P.; Huang, H.; Davis, M.; Calame, K.; Hood, L.: An immunoglobulin heavy chain variable region is generated from three segments of DNA: V_H, D, and J_H. Cell *19:* 981 (1980).

10 Kurosawa, Y.; Tonegawa, S.: Organization, structure and assembly of immunoglobulin heavy chain diversity DNA segments. J. exp. Med. *155:* 201 (1982).

11 Tonegawa, S.: Somatic generation of antibody diversity. Nature, Lond. *302:* 575 (1983).

12 Leder, P.: Genetic control of immunoglobulin production. Hosp. Pract. *18:* 73 (1983).

13 Honjo, T.; Habu, S.: Origin of immune diversity: genetic variation and selection. A. Rev. Biochem. *54:* 803 (1985).

14 Dildrop, R.: A new classification of mouse V_H sequences. Immunol. Today *5:* 85 (1984).

15 Brodeur, P.H.; Riblet, R.: The immunoglobulin heavy chain variable region (IgG-V) locus in the mouse. I. One hundred IgG-V genes comprise seven families of homologous genes. Eur. J. Immunol. *14:* 922 (1984).

16 Cory, S.; Tyler, B.M.; Adams, S.M.: Sets of immunoglobulin V kappa genes homologous to the cloned V kappa sequences. Implication for the number of germline V kappa genes. J. mol. appl. Genet. *1:* 103 (1981).

17 Livant, D.; Blatt, C.; Hood, L.: One heavy chain variable region gene segment subfamily in the BALB/c mouse contains 500–1,000 or more members. Cell *47:* 461 (1986).

18 Seidman, J.G.; Max, E.E.; Leder, P.: A K-immunoglobulin gene is formed by site-specific recombination without further somatic mutation. Nature, Lond. *280:* 370 (1979).

19 Swan, D.P.; D'Eustachio, P.; Leinwand, L.; Seidman, J.; Keithley, D.; Ruddle, F.H.: Chromosomal assignment of the mouse K light chain genes. Proc. natn. Acad. Sci. USA *76:* 2735 (1979).

20 D'Eustachio, P.; Bothwell, A.L.M.; Takaro, T.K.; Baltimore, D.; Ruddle, F.N.: Chromosomal location of structural genes encoding murine immunoglobulin λ light chains. J. exp. Med. *153:* 793 (1981).

21 Kindt, T.J.; Capra, J.D.: The antibody enigma (Plenum Press, New York 1984).

22 Alexander, A.; Rosen, S.; Buxbaum, J.: Human immunoglobulin genes in health and disease. Clin. Immunol. Rev. *4:* 31 (1985).

23 Potter, M.; Newell, J.B.; Rudikoff, S.; Haber, E.: Classification of mouse V_k groups based on the partial amino acid sequence to the first invariant tryptophan: Impact of 14 new sequences from IgG myeloma proteins. Molec. Immunol. *19:* 1619 (1982).

24 D'Hoostelaere, L.A.; Huppi, K.; Mock, B.; Mallett, C.; Potter, M.: The IgG haplotypes and IgK crossover populations suggest a gene order. J. Immun. *141:* 652 (1988).

25 Heller, M.; Owens, J.O.; Mushinski, J.F.; Rudikoff, S.: Amino acids at the site of V_K-J_K recombination not encoded by germline sequences. J. exp. Med. *166:* 638 (1987).

26 Alt, F.W.; Baltimore, D.: Joining of immunoglobulin heavy chain gene segments. Implications from a chromosome with evidence of three D-J_H fusions. Proc. natn. Acad. Sci. USA *79:* 4118 (1982).

27 Landau, N.R.; Shatz, D.G.; Rosa, M.; Baltimore, D.: Increased frequency of N-region insertion in a murine pre-B-cell line infected with a terminal deoxynucleotidyl transferase retroviral expression vector. Mol. cell. Biol. *7:* 3237 (1987).

28 Milstein, C.: From antibody structure to immunological diversification of immune response. Science *231:* 1261 (1986).

29 Kim, S.; Davis, M.; Sinn, E.; Pattern, P.; Hood, L.: Antibody diversity: somatic hypermutation of rearranged V_H genes. Cell *27:* 573 (1981).

30 Schiff, C.; Milili, M.; Fougereau, M.: Functional and pseudogenes are similarly organized and may equally contribute to the extensive antibody diversity of the Ig V_HII family. Eur. molec. Biol. Org. J. *4:* 1225 (1985).

31 Reynaud, C.; Anquez, V.; Dahan, A.; Weill, J.: A single rearrangement event generates most of the chicken immunoglobulin light chain diversity. Cell *40:* 283 (1985).

32 Reth, M.; Gehrmann, P.; Petrac, E.; Wiese, P.: A novel V_H to V_H DJ_H joining mechanism in heavy-chain-negative (null) pre-B cells results in heavy-chain production. Nature, Lond. *322:* 840 (1986).

33 Kleinfield, R.; Hardy, R.R.; Tarlinton, D.; Danyl, J.; Herzenberg, L.A.; Weigert, M.: Recombination between an expressed immunoglobulin heavy chain and a germline variable gene segment in a Ly 1+ B cell lymphoma. Nature, Lond. *322:* 843 (1986).

34 Krawinkel, U.; Zoebelin, G.; Bruggemann, M.; Radbruch, A.; Rajewsky, K.: Recombination between antibody heavy chain variable region genes: evidence for gene conversion. Proc. natn. Acad. Sci. USA *80:* 4997 (1983).

35 Thompson, C.B.; Neiman, P.E.: Somatic diversification of the chicken immunoglobulin light chain gene is limited to the rearranged variable segment. Cell *48:* 369 (1987).

36 Reynaud, C.-A.; Angvez, V.; Grimal, H.; Weill, J.-C.: A hyperconversion mechanism generates the chicken light chain preimmune repertoire. Cell *48:* 379 (1987).

37 Wabl, M.; Burrows, P.D.; Gabain, A. von; Steinberg, C.: Hypermutation of the human immunoglobulin heavy chain locus in a pre-B cell line. Proc. natn. Acad. Sci. USA *82:* 479 (1985).

38 Sablitzky, F.; Wildner, G.; Rajewsky, K.: Somatic mutation and clonal expansion of B cells in an antigen-driven immune response. Eur. molec. Biol. Org. J. *4:* 345 (1985).

39 Griffiths, G.M.; Berek, C.; Kaartinen, M.; Milstein, C.: Somatic mutation and the maturation of immune response to 2-phenyl oxazolone. Nature, Lond. *312:* 271 (1984).

40 McKean, D.; Huppi, K.; Bell, M.; Standt, L.; Gerhard, W.; Weigert, M.: Generation of antibody diversity in the immune response of BALB/c mice to influenza virus hemagglutinin. Proc. natn. Acad. Sci. USA *81:* 3180 (1984).

41 Clarke, S.H.; Huppi, K.; Ruezinsky, D.; Staudt, L.; et al.: Inter- and intraclonal diversity in the antibody response to influenza hemagglutinin. J. exp. Med. *161:* 687 (1985).

42 Clarke, S.H.; Rudikoff, S.: Evidence for gene conversion among immunoglobulin heavy chain variable region genes. J. exp. Med. *159:* 773 (1984).

43 Ferguson, S.E.; Rudikoff, S.; Osborne, B.A.: Interaction and sequence diversity among T15 V_H genes in CBA/J mice. J. exp. Med. *168:* 1339 (1988).

44 Rechavi, G.; Ram, D.; Glazer, L.; Zakut, R.; Givol, D.: Evolutionary aspects of immunoglobulin heavy chain variable region (V_H) gene subgroups. Proc. natn. Acad. Sci. USA *80:* 855 (1983).

45 Kodaira, M.; Kinashi, T.; Umemura, I.; Matsuda, F.; et al.: Organization and evolution of variable region genes of the human immunoglobulin heavy chain. J. molec. Biol. *190:* 529 (1986).

46 Diamond, B.A.; Scharff, M.D.: Somatic mutation of the T15 heavy chain genes give rise to an antibody with autoantibody specificity. Proc. natn. Acad. Sci. USA *81:* 5841 (1984).

47 Radbruch, A.; Zaiss, S.; Kappen, L.; Bruggemann, M.; Beyreuther, K.; Rajewsky, K.: Drastic change in idiotypic but not antigen-binding specificity of an antibody by a single amino acid substitution. Nature, Lond. *315:* 506 (1985).

48 Manser, T.; Gefter, M.L.: The molecular evolution of the immune response: idiotope specific suppression indicates that B cells express germ-line-encoded V genes prior to antigenic stimulation. Eur. J. Immunol. *16:* 1439 (1986).

49 Siekevitz, M.; Koch, C.; Rajewsky, K.; Dildrop, R.: Analysis of somatic mutation and class switching in naive and memory B cells generating adoptive primary and secondary responses. Cell *48:* 757 (1987).

50 Crews, S.; Griffin, J. Huang, H.; Calame, K.; Hood, L.: A single V_H gene segment encodes the immune response to phosphorylcholine: Somatic mutation is correlated with the class of antibody. Cell *25:* 59 (1981).

51 Koch, C.; Rajewsky, K.: Stepwise intraclonal maturation of antibody affinity through somatic mutation. Proc. natn. Acad. Sci. USA *85:* 8206 (1988).

52 Malipiero, U.V.; Levy, N.S.; Gearhart, P.J.: Somatic mutation in anti-phosphoryl-choline antibodies. Immunol. Rev. *96:* 59 (1987).

53 Berek, C.; Milstein, C.: Mutational drift and repertoire shift in the maturation of the immune response. Immunol. Rev. *96:* 23 (1987).

54 Manser, T.; Wysocki, L.J.; Margolies, M.N.; Gefter, M.L.: Evolution of antibody variable region structure during the immune response. Immunol. Rev. *96:* 141 (1987).

55 Allen, D.; Cumano, A.; Dildrop, R.; Koch, C.; Rajewsky, K.; et al.: Timing, genetic requirements, and functional consequences of somatic hypermutation during B-cell development. Immunol. Rev. *96:* 5 (1987).

56 Chien, N.C.; Pollock, R.R.; Desmayard, C.; Scharff, M.D.: Point mutations cause the somatic diversification of IgM and IgG anti-phosphorylcholine antibodies. J. exp. Med. *167:* 954 (1988).

57 Rudikoff, S.; Pawlita, M.; Pumphrey, J.; Heller, M.: Somatic diversification of immunoglobulins. Proc. natn. Acad. Sci. USA *81:* 2162 (1984).

58 Davidson, A.; Preud'homme, J.L.; Solomon, G.; Chang, M.-D.; Beede, S.; Diamond, B.: Idiotypic analysis of myeloma proteins: Anti-DNA activity of monoclonal immunoglobulins bearing an SLE idiotype is more common in IgG than IgM antibodies. J. Immun. *138:* 1515 (1987).

59 Kabat, E.A.; Wu, T.T.: Attempts to locate complementarity determining residues in the variable positions of light and heavy chains. Ann. N.Y. Acad. Sci. *190:* 382 (1971).

60 Poljak, R.J.; Anzel, L.M.; Avey, H.P.; Chen, B.L.; et al.: Three dimensional structure of the Fab' fragment of a human immunoglobulin at 2.8 A. Proc. natn. Acad. Sci. USA *70:* 3440 (1973).

61 Shlomchik, M.J.; Marshak-Rothstein, A.; Wolfowicz, C.B.; Rothstein, T.L.; Weigert, M.G.: The role of clonal selection and somatic mutation in autoimmunity. Nature, Lond. *328:* 805 (1987).

62 Riblet, R.; Brodeur, P.H.: The IgV_H gene repertoire in the mouse. Mount Sinai J. Med. *53:* 170 (1986).

63 Dildrop, R.; Bruggemann, M.; Radbruch, A.; Rajewsky, K.; Beyreuther, K.: Immunoglobulin V region variants in hybridoma cells II. Recombination between V genes. Eur. molec. Biol. Org. J. *1:* 635 (1981).

64 Kemp, D.J.; :Tyler, B.; Bernard, O.; Goush, N.; Gerondakis, S.; Adams, J.M.; Lory, S.: Organization of genes and spacers within the mouse immunoglobulin V_H locus. J. mol. appl. Genet. *1:* 245 (1981).

65 Schroeder, H.W., Jr.; Hillsohn, J.L.; Perlmutter, R.M.: Early restriction of the human antibody repertoire. Science *238:* 791 (1987).

66 Yancopoulos, G.D.; Malynn, B.A.; Alt, F.W.: Developmentally regulated and strain-specific expression of murine V_H families. J. exp. Med. *168:* 417 (1988).

67 Berman, J.; Mellis, S.; Pollack, R.; Smith, C.; Suh, H.Y.; Kowal, C.; Surti, U.; Chess, L.; Cantor, C.; Alt, F.: Content and organization of the human Ig V_H locus. Definition of three new V_H families and linkage to the Ig C_H locus. Eur. molec. Biol. Org. J. *7:* 727 (1988).

68 Sanz, I.: Hwang, L.Y.; Hasemann, C.; Thomas, J.; Wasserman, R.; Tucker, P.; Capra, J.D.: Polymorphisms of immunologically relevant loci in human disease: autoimmunity and human heavy chain variable regions. Ann. N.Y. Acad. Sci. (in press, 1988).

69 Jaenichen, H.R.; Pech, M.; Lindenmaier, W.; Weldgruber, N.; Zachau, H.G.: Composite human V_K genes and a model of their evolution. Nucl. Acids Res. *12:* 5249 (1984).

70 Klobeck, H.G.; Solomon, A.; Zachau, H.G.: Contribution of human V_K II germline genes to light chain diversity. Nature, Lond. *309:* 73 (1984).

71 Klobeck, H.G.; Meindl, A.; Combriato, G.; Solomon, A.; Zachau, H.G.: Human immunoglobulin kappa light chain genes of subgroups II and III. Nucl. Acids Res. *13:* 6499 (1985).

72 Klobeck, H.G.; Bornkamm, G.W.; Cambriato, G.; Mocikat, R.; Pohlenz, H.D.; Zachau, H.G.: Subgroup IV of human immunoglobulin K light chains is encoded by a single germline gene. Nucl. Acids Res. *13:* 6515 (1985).

73 Koffler, D.: Immunopathogenesis of systemic lupus erythematosus. A. Rev. Med. *25:* 149 (1984).

74 Williams, R.C., Jr.: Antibodies in systemic lupus – diversity finally simplified. J. Lab. clin. Med. *100:* 161 (1982).

75 Pisetsky, D.S.: Hybridoma SLE autoantibodies. Insights for the pathogenesis of autoimmune disease. Clin. Immunol. Rev. *3:* 169 (1984).

76 Dang, H.; Fischbach, M.; Lerner, E.; Talal, N.: Molecular and antigenic nature of isolated Sm. J. Immun. *130:* 2782 (1983).

77 Lerner, M.R.; Steitz, J.A.: Snurps and scyrps. Cell *25:* 298 (1981).

78 Lerner, M.R.; Steitz, J.A.: Antibodies to small nuclear RNAs complexed with protein are produced by patients with systemic lupus erythematosus. Proc. natn. Acad. Sci. USA *76:* 5495 (1979).

79 Bunn, C.C.; Gharavi, A.E.; Hughes, G.R.: Antibodies to extractable nuclear antigens in 173 patients with DNA-binding positive SLE. An association between antibodies to ribonucleoprotein and Sm antigens observed by counter immunoelectrophoresis. J. clin. Lab. Immunol. *8:* 13 (1982).

80 Yamagata, H.; Harley, J.B.; Reichlin, M.: Molecular properties of the Ro/SSA antigen and enzyme-linked immunosorbent assay for quantitation of antibody. J. clin. Invest. *74:* 625 (1984).

81 Harley, J.B.; Yamagata, H.; Reichlin, M.: Anti-La/SSB antibody is present in some normal sera and is coincident with anti-Ro/SSA precipitins in systemic lupus erythematosus. J. Rheumatol. *11:* 309 (1984).

82 Stollar, B.D.: Antibodies to DNA. CRC Rev. Biochem. *20:* 1 (1986).

83 Stollar, D.; Levine, L.; Lehrer, H.I.; Van Vounaki, H.: The antigenic determinants of denatured DNA reactive with lupus erythematosus serum. Proc. natn. Acad. Sci. USA *48:* 874 (1962).

84 Emlen, W.; Pisetsky, D.S.; Taylor, R.P.: Antibodies to DNA. A perspective. Arthritis Rheum. *29:* 1417 (1986).

85 Casperson, G.F.; Voss, E.W., Jr.: Specificity of anti-DNA antibodies in SLE II. Relative contribution of backbone, secondary structure and nucleotide sequence to DNA binding. Molec. Immunol. *20:* 58 (1983).

86 Schwartz, R.S.; Stollar, B.D.: Origins of anti-DNA antibodies. J. clin. Invest. *75:* 321 (1985).

87 Andre-Schwartz, J.; Datta, S.K.; Schoenfeld, Y.; Isenberg, D.A.; Stollar, B.D.; Schwartz, R.S.: Binding of cytoskeletal proteins by monoclonal anti-DNA lupus antibodies. Clin. Immunol. Immunopathol. *31:* 261 (1984).

88 Rauch, J.; Tannenbaum, H.; Stollar, B.D.; Schwartz, R.S.: Monoclonal anti-cardiolipin antibodies bind to DNA. Eur. J. Immunol. *14:* 529 (1984).

89 Jacob, L.; Tron, F.; Bach, J.-F.; Louvard, D.: A monoclonal anti-DNA antibody also binds cell surface proteins. Proc. natn. Acad. Sci. USA *81:* 3843 (1984).

90 Theofilopoulos, A.N.; Dixon, F.J.: Murine models of systemic lupus erythematosus. Adv. Immunol. *37:* 269 (1985).

91 Rosenburg, Y.J.; Steinberg, A.D.; Santoro, T.J.: The basis of autoimmunity in MRL/ 1pr mice. A role for self Ia-reactive T cells. Immunol. Today *5:* 64 (1984).

92 Wofsky, D.; Ledbetter, J.A.; Hendler, P.L.; Seaman, W.E.: Treatment of murine lupus with monoclonal anti-T cell antibody. J. Immun. *134:* 852 (1985).

93 Wofsy, D.; Seaman, W.E.: Successful treatment of autoimmunity in NZB/NZW F1 mice with monoclonal antibody to L3T4. J. exp. Med. *161:* 378 (1985).

94 Wofsy, D.; Seaman, W.E.: Reversal of advanced murine lupus in NZB/NZW F1 mice by treatment with monoclonal antibody to L3T4. J. Immun. *138:* 3247 (1987).

95 Shirai, T.; Hivose, S.; Sekigawa, I.; Okada, T.; Sato, H.: Genetic and cellular basis of anti-DNA antibody synthesis in systemic lupus erythematosus in New Zealand mice. J. Rheumatol. *14:* (suppl. 13, pp. 11–20 (1987).

96 Ando, D.G.; Sercarz, E.E.; Hahn, B.H.: Mechanisms of T and B cell collaboration in the in vitro production of anti-DNA antibodies in the NZB/NZW F1 muring SLE model. J. Immun. *138:* 3185 (1987).

97 Klinman, D.M.; Steinberg, A.D.: Systemic autoimmune disease arises from polyclonal B-cell activation. J. exp. Med. *165:* 1755 (l1987).

98 Klinman, D.M.; Steinberg, A.D.: Proliferation of anti-DNA producing NZB B cells in a non-autoimmune environment. J. Immun. *137:* 69 (1986).

99 Shoenfeld, Y.; Vilner, Y.; Coates, A.R.M.; Rauch, J.; et al.: Monoclonal antituberculosis antibodies react with DNA and monoclonal anti-DNA autoantibodies react with *Mycobacterium tuberculosis*. Clin. exp. Immunol. *66:* 103 (1986).

100 Carroll, P.; Stafford, D.; Schwartz, R.S.; Stollar, B.D.: Murine monoclonal anti-DNA autoantibodies bind to endogenous bacteria. J. Immun. *135:* 1086 (1985).

101 Kabat, E.A.; Nickerson, K.G.; Liao, J.; Grossbard, L.; et al.: A human monoclonal macroglobulin with specificity for alpha C2-8 linked poly-N-acetyl neuraminic acid, the capsular polysaccharide of group B meningocci and *Escherichia coli* K1, which cross reacts with polynucleotides an denatured DNA. J. exp. Med. *164:* 642 (1986).

102 Hoch, S.; Schur, P.H.; Schwaber, J.: Frequency of anti-DNA producing cells from normals and patients with systemic lupus erythematosus. Clin. Immunol. Immunopathol. *27:* 28 (1983).

103 Cairns, E.; Block, J.; Bell, D.A.: Anti-DNA autoantibody producing hybridomas of normal human lymphoid cell origin. J. clin. Invest. *74:* 880 (1984).

104 Hoch, S.; Schwaber, J.: Specificity analysis of human anti-DNA antibodies. J. Immun. *136:* 892 (1986).

105 Schoenfeld, Y.; Rauch, J.; Maniscotte, H.; Datta, S.K.; Andre-Schwartz, J.; Stollar, B.D.; Schwartz, R.S.: Polyspecificity of monoclonal lupus autoantibodies produced by human-human hybridomas. New Engl. J. Med. *308:* 414 (1983).

106 Madaio, M.P.; Schattner, A.; Schattner, M.; Schwartz, R.S.: Lupus serum and normal human serum with the same idiotypic marker. J. Immun. *137:* 2535 (1986).

107 Naparstek, Y.; André-Schwartz, J.; Manser, T.; Wysocki, L.; Breitman, L.; et al.: A single germline V_H gene segment of normal A/J mice encodes autoantibodies characteristic of systemic lupus erythematosus. J. exp. Med. *164:* 614 (1986).

108 Schoenfeld, Y.; Hsu-Lin, S.C.; Gabrices, J.E.; Silberstein, L.E.; Furie, B.C.; et al.: Production of autoantibodies by human-human hybridomas. J. clin. Invest. *70:* 205 (1982).

109 Rauch, J.; Maniscotte, H.; Tannebaum, H.: Hybridoma anti-DNA autoantibodies from patients with rheumatoid arthritis and systemic lupus erythematosus demonstrate similar nucleic acid binding characteristics. J. Immun. *134:* 180 (1985).

110 Avrameas, S.: Natural autoreactive B cells and autoantibodies: the 'know thyself' of the immune system. Annals Inst. Pasteur/Immunol., Paris *137D:* 149 (1986).

111 Nakamura, M.; Burastero, S.E.; Ueki, Y.; Larrick, J.W.; Notkins, A.L.; Casali, P.: Probing the normal and autoimmune B cell repertoire with Epstein-Barr virus. Frequency of B cells producing monoreactive high affinity autoantibodies in patients with Hashimoto's disease and systemic lupus erythematosus. J. Immun. *141:* 4165 (1988).

112 Lafer, E.M.; Rauch, J.; Andrzejewski, C.; Mudd, D.; Furie, B.C.; et al.: Polyspecific monoclonal lupus autoantibodies reactive with polynucleotides and phospholipids. J. exp. Med. *153:* 897 (1981).

113 Rubin, R.L., Balderaas, R.S., Tan, E.M.; Dixon, F.J.; Theofiloplous, A.N.: Multiple autoantigen binding capabilities of mouse monoclonal antibodies selected for rheumatoid factor activity. J. exp. Med. *159:* 1429 (1984).

114 Davidson, A.; Smith, A.; Katz, J.; Preud'homme, J.L.; Solomon, A.; Diamond, B.: A cross reactive idiotype on anti-DNA antibodies may be somatically generated and antigen driven (submitted).

115 Jerne, N.K.: Idiotypic networks and other preconceived ideas. Immunol. Rev. *79:* 5 (1984).

116 Isenberg, D.A.; Schoenfeld, :Y.; Madaio, M.P.; Rauch, J.; Reichlin, M.; Stollar, B.D.; Schwartz, R.S.: Anti-DNA antibody idiotypes in systemic lupus erythematosus. Lancet *ii:* 417 (1984).

117 Rauch, J.; Mansicotte, H.; Tannenbaum, H.: Specified and shared idiotypes found on hybridoma anti-DNA autoantibodies derived from rheumatoid arthritis and systemic lupus erythematosus patients. J. Immun. *135:* 2385 (1985).

118 Isenberg, D.A.; Dudeney, C.; Wojnaruska, F.; Bhogal, B.S.; Rauch, J.; Schattner, A.; Naparstek, Y.; Duggan, D.: Detection of cross reactive anti-DNA antibody idiotypes

on tissue bound-immunoglobulins from skin biopsies of lupus patients. J. Immun. *135:* 261 (1985).

119 Morgan, A.; Isenberg, D.A.; Naparstek, Y.; Rauch, J.; Duggan, D.; Khiroya, R.; Staines, N.A.; Schattner, A.: Shared idiotypes are expressed on mouse and human anti-DNA autoantibodies. Immunology *56:* 393 (1985).

120 Essani, K.; Satoh, J.; Prabhakar, B.S.; McClintoh, P.R.; Notkins, A.L.: Anti-idiotypic antibodies against a human multiple organ-reactive autoantibody. J. clin. Invest. *76:* 1649 (1985).

121 Halpern, R.; Schiffenbauer, J.; Solomon, G.; Diamond, B.: Detection of masked anti-DNA antibodies in lupus sera by a monoclonal anti-idiotype. J. Immun. *133:* 1852 (1984).

122 Valesini, G.; Tincani, A.; Harris, E.N.; Mantelli, P.G.; Allegri, F.; Palmieri, F.; Hughes, G.R.; Balsano, F.; Ballestrieri, G.: Use of monoclonal antibodies to identify shared idiotypes on anti-cardiolipin and anti-DNA antibodies in human sera. Clin. exp. Immunol. *69:* 1 (1987).

123 Eilat, D.; Fischel, R.; Zlotnick, A.: A central anti-DNA idiotype in human and murine systemic lupus erythematosus. Eur. J. Immunol. *15:* 368 (1985).

124 Aguis, M.; Richman, D.: Suppression of development of experimental autoimmune myasthenia gravis with isogenic monoclonal anti-idiotypic antibody. J. Immun. *137:* 2195 (1986).

125 Zouali, M.; Fine, J.M.; Eyquem, A.: Anti-DNA autoantibody activity and idiotypic relationships of human monoclonal proteins. Eur. J. Immunol. *14:* 1085 (1984).

126 Solomon, G.; Schiffenbauer, J.; Keiser, H.; Diamond, B.: Use of monoclonal antibodies to identify shared idiotypes on human antibodies to native DNA from patients with systemic lupus erythematosus. Proc. natn. Acad. Sci. USA *80:* 850 (1983).

127 Bell, D.A.; Cairns, E.; Cikalo, K.; Ly, V.; Block, J.; Pruzanski, W.: Anti-nucleic acid autoantibody responses of normal human origin: antigen specificity and idiotypic characteristics compared to patients with systemic lupus erythematosus and patients with monoclonal IgM. J. Rheumatol. *14:* 127 (1987).

128 Livneh, A.; Halpern, A.; Perkins, D.; Lazo, A.; Halpern, R.; Diamond, B.: A monoclonal antibody to a cross-reactive idiotype on cationic human anti-DNA antibodies expressing lambda light chains: a new reagent to identify a potentially differential pathogenic subset. J. Immun. *138:* 123 (1987).

129 Takei, M.; Dang, H.; Talal, N.: A common idiotype expressed on a murine anti-Sm monoclonal antibody and antibodies in SLE sera. Clin. exp. Immunol. *70:* 546 (1987).

130 Naparstek, Y.; Duggan, D.; Schattner, A.; Madaio, M.; Goni, F.; Frangione, B.; Stollar, D.; Kabat, E.; Schwartz, R.S.: Immunochemical similarities between monoclonal antibacterial Waldenstrom's macroglobulins and monoclonal anti-DNA lupus autoantibodies. J. exp. Med. *161:* 1525 (1985).

131 Mackworth-Young, C.; Sabbaga, J.; Schwartz, R.S.: Idiotypic markers of polyclonal B cell activation. Public idiotypes shared by monoclonal antibodies derived from patients with systemic lupus erythematosus and leprosy. J. clin. Invest. *79:* 572 (1987).

132 Williams, W.; Zumla, A.; Behrens, R.; Locniskar, M.; Voller, A.; McAdam, K.P.W.J.; Isenberg, D.A.: Studies of a common idiotype PR4 in autoimmune rheumatic disease. Arthritis Rheum. *31:* 1097 (1988).

133 Bellon, B.; Manheimer-Lory, A.; Monestier, M.; Moran, T.; Dimitriu-Bona, A.; Alt F.; Bona, C.: High frequency of autoantibodies bearing cross reactive idiotypes among hybridomas using V_H 7183 genes from normal and autoimmune animals. J. clin. Invest. *79:* 1044 (1987).

134 Chen, P.P.; Liu, M.F.; Sinha, S.; Carson, D.: A 16/16 idiotype positive anti-DNA antibody is encoded by a conserved V_H gene with no somatic mutation. Arthritis Rheum. *31:* 1429 (1988).

135 Chen, P.P.; Goni, F.; Fong, S.; Jirik, F.; Vaughan, J.H.; Frangione, B.; Carson, D.A.: The majority of human monoclonal IgM rheumatoid factors express a 'primary-structure dependent' cross-reactive idiotype. J. Immun. *134:* 3281 (1985).

136 Isenberg, D.A.; Collins, C.: Detection of cross-reactive anti-DNA antibody idiotypes on renal tissue bound immunoglobulins from lupus patients. J. clin. Invest. *76:* 287 (1985).

137 Isenberg, D.A.; Schoenfeld, Y.; Walport, C.; Mackworth-Young, C.; et al.: Detection of cross-reactive anti-DNA antibody idiotypes on the serum of systemic lupus erythematosus patients and of their relatives. Arthritis Rheum. *28:* 999 (1985).

138 Andrzejewski, C., Jr.; Rauch, J.; Lafer, F.; Stollar, B.D.; Schwartz, R.S.: Antigen-binding diversity and idiotypic cross-reaction, among hybridoma autoantibodies to DNA. J. Immun. *126:* 226 (1981).

139 Rauch, J.; Murphy, E.; Roths, J.B.; Stollar, B.D.; Schwartz, R.S.: A high frequency idiotypic marker of anti-DNA autoantibodies in MRL/lpr mice. J. Immun. *129:* 236 (1982).

140 Datta, S.K.; Stollar, B.D.; Schwartz, R.S.: Normal mice express idiotypes related to autoantibody idiotypes of lupus mice. Proc. natn. Acad. Sci. USA *80:* 2723 (1983).

141 Hahn, B.H.; Ebling, F.M.: Suppression of murine lupus nephritis by administration of an anti-idiotypic antibody to anti-DNA. J. Immun. *132:* 187 (1984).

142 Marion, T.N.; Lawton, A.R. III; Kearney, J.F.; Briles, D.E.: Anti-DNA autoantibodies in (NZB×NZW) F1 mice are clonally heterogeneous but the majority share a common idiotype. J. Immun. *128:* 668 (1982).

143 Tron, F.; Jacob, L.; Bach, J.F.: Murine monoclonal anti-DNA idiotypes with an absolute specificity for DNA have a large amount of idiotypic diversity. Proc. natn. Acad. Sci. USA *80:* 6024 (1983).

144 Hahn, B.A.; Ebling, F.M.: A public idiotype determinant is present on spontaneous cationic IgG antibodies to DNA from mice of unrelated lupus-prone strains. J. Immun. *133:* 3015 (1984).

145 Hahn, B.H.; Ebling, F.M.: Idiotype restriction in murine lupus; high frequency of three idiotypes on serum IgG in nephritic NZB/NZW F1 mice. J. Immun. *138:* 2110 (1987).

146 Halpern, R.; Davidson, A.; Lazo, A.; Solomon, G.; Lahita, R.; Diamond, B.: Familial systemic lupus erythematosus. Presence of a cross-reactive idiotype in healthy family members. J. clin. Invest. *76:* 731 (1985).

147 Ebling, F.; Hahn, B.: Restricted subpopulations of DNA antibodies in kidneys of mice with systemic lupus. Arthritis Rheum. *23:* 392 (1980).

148 El-Roiey, A.; Sela, O.; Isenberg, D.A.; Feldman, R.; Colaco, B.C.; Kennedy, R.C.; Schoenfeld, Y.: The sera of patients with Klebsiella infections contain a common anti-DNA idiotype (16/6) Id and antipolynucleotide activity. Clin. exp. Immunol. *67:* 507 (1987).

149 Isenberg, D.A.; Colaco, C.B.; Dudeney, C.; Todd-Pokropeck, A.; Smith, M.L.: The relationship of anti-DNA antibody idiotypes and anticardiolipin antibodies to disease activity in systemic lupus erythematosus. Medicine 65: 46 (1986).

150 Harris, E.N.; Gharavi, A.E.; Tincani, A.; Chan, J.K.; Englert, H.; Mantelli, P.; Allegro, F.; Ballestrieri, G.; Hughes, G.: Affinity purified anti-cardiolipin antibodies and anti-DNA antibodies. J. clin. Lab. Immunol. 17: 155 (1985).

151 Lafer, E.M.; Rauch, J.; Andrezejewski, C.; Mudd, D.; Furie, B.; Schwartz, R.S.; Stollar, B.D.: Polyspecific monoclonal lupus autoantibodies reactive with both polynucleotides and phospholipids. J. exp. Med. 152: 897 (1981).

152 Dersimonian H.; Schwartz, R.S.; Barrett, K.; Stollar, B.D.: Relationship of human variable region heavy chain germ line genes to genes encoding anti-DNA autoantibodies. J. Immun. 139: 2496 (1987).

153 Roubinian; Papoian; Talal, N.: Effects of neonatal thymectomy on survival and regulation of autoantibody formation in NZB/NZW F_1 mice. J. Immun. 118: 1524 (1977).

154 Davidson, A.; Shefner, R.; Livneh, A.; Diamond, B.: The role of somatic mutation of immunoglobulin genes in autoimmunity. A. Rev. Immunol. 5: 85 (1987).

155 Madaio, M.P.; Schattner, A.; Shattner, M.; Schwartz, R.S.: Lupus serum and normal human serum contain anti-DNA antibodies with the same idiotypic marker. J. Immun. 137: 2535 (1986).

156 Query, C.C.; Keene, J.D.: A human autoimmune protein associated with U1 RNA contains a region of homology that is cross reactive with retroviral p30 gag antigen. Cell 51: 211 (1987).

157 Rechavi, G.; Bienz, B.; Ram, D.; Ben-Neviah, Y.; Cohen, J.B.; et al.: Organization and evolution of immunoglobulin V_H gene subgroups. Proc. natn. Acad. Sci. USA 79: 4405 (1982).

158 Arant, S.E.; Griffin, J.A.; Koopman, E.J.: V_H gene expression is restricted in anti-IgG antibodies from MRL autoimmune mice. J. exp. Med. 164: 1284 (1986).

159 Aguado, M.Y.; Balderas, R.S.; Rubin, R.L.; Duchosal, M.A.; et al.: Specificity and molecular characteristics of monoclonal IgM rheumatoid factors from arthritic and non-arthritic mice. J. Immun. 139: 1080 (1987).

160 Monestier, M. Manheimer-Lory, A.; Bellon, B.; Painter, C.; et al.: Shared idiotypes and restricted immunoglobulin variable region heavy chain genes characterize murine autoantibodies of various specificities. J. clin. Invest. 78: 753 (1986).

161 Dighiero, G.; Lymberi, P.; Holmberg, D.; Lindquist, I.; Coutinho, A.; Avrameas, S.: High frequency of natural autoantibodies in normal newborn mice. J. Immun. 131: 2267 (1985).

162 Shlomchik, J.M.; Nemazee, D.; Van Snick, J.; Weigert, M.: Variable region sequences of murine IgM anti-IgG monoclonal autoantibodies (rheumatoid factors). II. Comparison of hybridomas derived by lipopolysaccharide stimulation and secondary protein immunization. J. exp. Med. 165: 970 (1987).

163 Shlomchik, J.M.; Nemazee, D.A.; Sato, V.L.; van Snick, J.; et al.: Variable region sequences of murine IgM anti-IgG monoclonal autoantibodies (rheumatoid factors). J. exp. Med. 164: 407 (1986).

164 Shlomchik, M.J.; Aucoin, A.H.; Pisetsky, D.S.; Weigert, M.G.: Structure and function of anti-DNA autoantibodies derived from a single autoimmune mouse. Proc. natn. Acad. Sci. USA 84: 9150 (1987).

165 Behar, S.M.; Scharff, M.D.: Somatic diversification of the S107 (T15) V_H11 germline gene that encodes anti-dsDNA Abs in (NZB/NZW) F1 mice. Proc. natn. Acad. Sci. USA *85:* 3970 (1988).

166 Eisenberg, R.A.; Winfield, J.B.; Cohen, P.C.: Subclass reconstruction of anti-Sm response in MRL mice. J. Immun. *129:* 2146 (1982).

167 Jerne, N.K.: Towards a network theory of the immune system. Ann. Immunol., Paris *125:* 373 (1974).

168 Schiff, C.; Milili, M.; Hue, I.; Rudikoff, S.; Fougereau, M.: Genetic bassis for expression of the idiotypic network. One unique Ig V_H germ line gene accounts for the major family of Ab1 and Ab3 (Ab1′) antibodies of the GAT system. J. exp. Med. *163:* 573 (1986).

169 Margolies, M.N.; Wysocki, L.J.; Sato, V.L.: Immunoglobulin idiotype and anti-anti-idiotype utilize the same variable region genes irrespective of antigen specificity. J. Immun. *130:* 515 (1983).

170 Reth, M.; Kelsoe, G.; Rajewsky, K.: Idiotypic regulation by isologous monoclonal anti-idiotype antibodies. Nature, Lond. *290:* 257 (1981).

171 Mendlovic, S.; Brocke, S.; Shoenfeld, Y.; Ben-Basset, M.; Meshorer, A.; Bakimer, R.; Mozes, E.: Induction of a systemic lupus erythematosus like disease in mice by a human anti-DNA idiotype. Proc. natn. Acad. Sci. USA *85:* 2260 (1988).

R. Shefner, MD, Albert Einstein College of Medicine,
1300 Morris Park Avenue, Bronx, NY 10461 (USA)

Carson DA, Chen PP, Kipps TJ (eds): Idiotypes in Biology and Medicine.
Chem Immunol. Basel, Karger, 1990, vol 48, pp 109–125

Cold Agglutinins: Specificity, Idiotypy and Structural Analysis[1]

Gregg J. Silverman, Pojen P. Chen, Dennis A. Carson

Department of Basic and Clinical Research, Research Institute of Scripps Clinic, La Jolla, Calif., USA

Introduction

Among the vast array of potential self antigens only a small number are the known targets of autoimmune attack. Cold agglutinins (CAs) are antibodies that bind to the surfaces of autologous erythrocytes, causing agglutination upon cooling. Although antibodies of similar specificity may occur in a variety of infectious and inflammatory responses, high concentrations of these antibodies most often occur in lymphoproliferative syndromes, chronic cold agglutinin disease, or as part of chronic lymphocytic leukemias and lymphomas [1]. Among human monoclonal IgM proteins, CAs and rheumatoid factors (RFs) (i.e. antibodies with anti-IgC Fc activity) are the most common autoantibodies, and each represents 5–10% of these proteins [12]. Study of these antibodies has allowed the characterization of red cell membrane structures, and enabled insights into the structural and genetic basis of immunoglobulin production.

Specificity and Immunochemistry

Antibodies that agglutinate erythrocytes in the cold may be directed against an array of membrane determinants. CAs are usually of the IgM isotype, and most are directed against the I/i system. The anti-I specificity is assigned if there is hemagglutination at 4 °C of adult O⁺ red cells at titers

[1] Funding for this research supported in part by grants A100866, AR25443, RR00833 and AR33489 from the National Institutes of Health.

fourfold or greater than with umbilical cord cells. If umbilical cells are preferentially bound, i specificity is assigned. Anti-I/i activity is retained after red cells are treated with protease [2].

Fukuda, Hakomori and others have demonstrated that anti-I antibodies are directed against a carbohydrate determinant on a glycoconjugate that is developmentally regulated [3, reviewed in 2, 4]. At birth the vast majority of these molecules are repeating N-acetyl lactosamine molecules, which express the i determinants. During the first 2 years of life an increasing proportion acquire a branched oligosaccharide structure, involved in the I determinants. These determinants also represent the precursors of the ABH and Lewis blood group substances [5, 6]. On red cells and B lymphocytes I determinants are expressed on glycolipids and glycoproteins, while in body fluids, such as plasma, saliva and milk, they are glycoproteins. Among monoclonal IgM CAs multiple distinct I and i epitopes may be recognized [6]. Antibodies with CA activity are present in the sera of normal adults and neonates, and anti-I antibodies represent the largest proportion [7]. Levels in normal subjects are highest in females, and correlate with secretor status [8].

Many inflammatory disorders may be associated with CAs as part of the polyclonal induction of immunoglobulins. In other disorders specific increases of these antibodies occur. Epitopes similar to those in I/i are present in type XIV pneumococcal polysaccharide. Antibodies to these bacterial capsule structures have been shown to exhibit in vitro CA-like activity [9]. Although autoimmune hemolysis is not a major aspect of clinical pneumococcal infection, CAs do occur in anemia of chronic malaria infection [10]. Also, drug-induced autoimmune hemolysis may involve the induction of antibodies to the I antigen on the surface of red cells [11].

The infectious agent most commonly associated with a specific induction CAs is *Mycoplasma pneumoniae*. Most patients with *M. pneumoniae* infection will develop these autoantibodies, and circulating erythrocytes become Coombs positive. However, significant hemolysis is uncommon [12]. Mycoplasma-induced CAs are polyclonal and often kappa restricted [13], although lambda L chains in these CAs have also been described [14]. In an experimental model, rabbits produced anti-I antibodies when immunized with human erythrocytes treated with Mycoplasma, while this did not occur after immunization with either Mycoplasma or red cells alone [15]. Mycoplasma may therefore induce cold agglutinin production by one of two possible mechanisms: (1) these antibodies may arise as part of a polyclonal B cell activation; or (2) Mycoplasma infection may interact with red cell surface structures, causing I epitopes that then become antigenic. In support of the latter, red cell I structures act as specific Mycoplasma receptors, which may then facilitate antigen presentation of I epitopes in an immunogenic form [15a].

Infectious mononucleosis caused by Epstein-Barr virus may cause a polyclonal B cell activation with production of CAs (as well as a multitude of other autoantibodies). These CA antibodies are also usually polyclonal, and are primarily directed against i determinants. Like monoclonal CAs against i, these antibodies most commonly use lambda L chains [16, 17]. Further, CA occurring during infectious mononucleosis are often of the IgG isotype. For this reason, circulating IgM rheumatoid factors (anti-IgG) may be required for the demonstration of cold-induced hemagglutination [18]. In other cases both IgG and IgM CAs are detected [19]. Infection-induced CAs may use similar V regions as monoclonal CAs, as these antibodies often share cross-reacting serologic reactivity (idiotypes) [20].

The Pr system represents a system of red cell associated determinants that is completely distinct from I/i. Anti-Pr specificity is demonstrated if hemagglutination is decreased or lost after treatment of red cells with protease. The Pr epitopes are now known to be present on a set of related linear glycoproteins which involves sialic acid [4, 21, 22]. Monoclonal antibodies against these epitopes are less common than those against the I/i system and are usually associated with lymphoproliferative disorders, although they may occur in infectious mononucleosis. These antibodies can be IgM, IgG or IgA isotype. Other uncommon specificities of cold agglutinating antibodies have been described, including the Donath Landsteiner antibody of paroxysmal nocturnal hemoglobinuria, and the anti-Gd (glycolipid dependent) and anti-Sa system [2, 23, 24].

Idiotypy and Anti-Pr CAs

The monoclonal CAs to Pr determinants use a set of L chains different from those used in anti-I CAs. Many anti-Pr L chains share cross-reactive determinants. In 1973 Wang [25] demonstrated that the L chains of two anti-Pr CAs had near-identical sequences. These L chains were different from other described kappa chains and they derive from a new subgroup, designated KIV. More recently, Zachau and co-workers have demonstrated that in the germline there is only one KIV gene. Further, within the Vk locus, this gene is most Jk proximal [26]. Yancopoulos et al. [27] have shown that in the mouse VH chain locus, genes most JH proximal are preferentially rearranged during early ontogeny. Similarly, the human KIV gene is preferentially rearranged in the fetal liver [Hillson, in preparation] and in lymphoid cell lines [28]. Whether anti-Pr CA autoantibodies are expressed due to this mechanism is unknown.

The H chains of anti-Pr CAs have long been known to share cross-reacting determinants unrelated to those in anti-I/i antibodies [29]. There is evidence that similar VH genes are used in anti-Pr CAs from unrelated individuals. Two partial and one complete H chain sequence have been reported, and these are all VHIII proteins, although there is inadequate data to suggest whether these derive from the same gene [30].

Anti-I CAs, Idiotypy and L Chain Use

Some of the earliest studies on idiotypes demonstrated cross-reactive determinants on anti-I CAs [31]. Monoclonal antibodies to I were later shown to be highly kappa L chain restricted [32]. The majority of these kappa L chains are structurally related and by serologic studies they often belong to the minor KIIIb sub-subgroup [33]. Few of these CAs use either KI or KII L chains [34]. Eight partial sequences of KIII anti-I CAs are displayed in comparison to the deduced amino acid sequence of the human kv325 germline gene (table 1) [34, 35]. Sequence comparison of these L chains suggests that they have greater structural homology to the germline Humkv325 gene, than to the 12 other described KIII genes [36]. While the kv325 gene is most closely linked to monoclonal RFs, L chains of antibodies to intermediate filaments, low density lipoprotein with complete, or near complete sequence identity to the deduced sequence of kv325 have also recently been described [37].

In an effort to obtain more information about the L chains used in anti-I CAs, a large collection of these proteins has been studied with peptide-induced antibodies. From the L chain of the kv325 derived RF, Sie, the sequence of a portion of the second complementarity-determining region (CDR) and adjacent framework region 3 (designated PSL2), and the sequence of the third CDR (designated PSL3) were used to make synthetic peptides (reviewed in RF companion chapter). After conjugation to keyhole limpet hemocyanin, antibodies to these primary sequences were then raised in rabbits, and designated anti-PSL2 and anti-PSL3, respectively [38]. As a complement to these kv325 gene product markers, a panel of more broadly reactive antipeptide antibodies was next developed. These antisera recognize

Table 1. Comparison of the kv325 germline sequence and the partial amino acid sequences of eight monoclonal cold agglutinins reported previously [34, 35, 61].

	1		4	CDR1 30A 4	
Humkv325	E IVLTQSPGT	LS LS PGERAT	LS CRASQS VS	SS YLAW YQQK	PGQAPRILLIY
Cold agglutinin K chains					
1 Joh (AJ)	-------D-	---------	----------	------	-----------
2 Dre	---------	------V-	----------	----	-----------
3 GJ	---------	------V-	---		-----------
4 Ma	---------	---------	----------		-----------
5 Nic	----Z----	-----Z-	----------		-----------
6 Per	---------	-----Z-	-----Z		-----------
7 Ste	----Z---	-----A	--		-----------
8 Tak	----Z---	---Z-V-	----------	X----	-----------
Germline Vk gene					
1 Humkv305	---------S-	---------	---G----	----------	--L----
2 Humkv328	--M----A-	--V-	----------	-N----	--------
3 Humkv3g	------A-	---------	----------	----------	--------
4 Humkv3h	--M----P-	---V-	----------	---T----	--------

The kv325 sequence is displayed in the one–letter code at top, and only variant residues are given below. Z represents either a glutamine or glutamic acid residue. X in Tak represents a residue which may be either Ser, Gly, or Trp. Other KIII germline sequences are depicted below [36], and these are unlikely origins of these CA L chains.

Table 2. Antipeptide reactivity with RF L chains

	49						55				60				Anti-PSL2 reactivity
PSL2	Y	G	A	S	S	R	A	T	G	I	P	D	R	(C)	
BOR	–	–	–	–	–	–	–	–	–	–	–	–	–		+
LES	–	–	–	–	T	–	–	–	–	–	–	A	–		WK
RIV	–	D	T	–	N	–	–	–	–	–	–	A	–		WK

Above these homologous portions of L chain variable region sequences is listed the residue number according to Kabat et al. [45]. The one-letter amino acid code is used, and the use of an identical residue is shown with (–). As demonstrated in figure 1, reactivity of each L chain with the anti-PSL2 reagent is listed as either strong (+) or weak (WK).

a diagnostic portion of kappa first framework regions. Each of these reagents recognizes only L chains from one of the four kappa subgroups, KI, KII, KIII and KIV (designated anti-PKI, anti-PKII, anti-PKIII and anti-PKIV, respectively) [39, 40].

A total of 13 anti-I CAs have now been studied with these reagents, of which 2 use KII and 11 use KIII L chains. To demonstrate the diagnostic specificity of the anti-KIII antiserum, many KIII L chains of known amino acid sequence have been studied and 21/22 are reactive [39, 40; unpubl. data]. Further, the KIII-specific antiserum is nonreactive with the 8 KI, 6 KII and 1 KIV L chains of known sequence that have been tested. By a similar analysis the anti-PSL3 reagent has been shown to identify only the products of the germline configuration of the kv325 gene (see companion chapter). To demonstrate the specificity of the anti-PSL2 reagent, portions of the amino acid sequence of 3 IgM RFs are displayed in juxtaposition to the peptide sequence used to induce the anti-PSL2 sera, in table 2. The binding activity of anti-PSL2 with these 3 RFs and 5 anti-I CAs is illustrated in figure 1. Among the RFs the strongest anti-PSL2 reactivity is against Bor, which in this region is identical to the PSL2 sequence. Bor is also reactive with anti-PSL3 and likely derives from the kv325 gene. The Les RF has only weak reactivity with anti-PSL2 and it varies by 2 residues from the PSL2 sequence. Similarly, the Les L chain is nonreactive with anti-PSL3, and sequence comparison suggests it may derive from Humkv328, a different germline gene [41]. The KIII-RF, Riv, reacts weakly with anti-PSL2 but not with anti-PSL3, and sequence comparison suggests that it may be derived from yet another KIII gene, which has not yet been isolated and characterized [42].

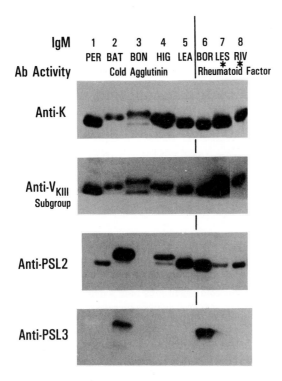

Fig. 1. Immunoblot analysis of the L chains of monoclonal IgM CAs and RFs. After SDS-PAGE separation and transfer to nitrocellulose, replicate blots of the L chains of five IgM CAs and three IgM RFs were reacted with the indicated antipeptide antibodies. The anti-K antiserum was derived with a sequence from the amino terminal end of the kappa constant region. (*) L chains are non-KIIIb and probably do not derive from the kv325 germline gene, based on sequence comparison. Adapted from Silverman et al. [49].

These data show that the anti-PSL2 identifies a subset of KIII proteins, and that anti-PSL2 in conjunction with anti-PSL3 identify kv325-derived proteins.

Extending this analysis to anti-I CAs, 4/11 (Bat, Kau, Pos, Tri) of the KIII CAs are identified as products of the kv325 gene as they bear the PSL2 and PSL3 markers (fig. 1; table 3). In addition, based on amino-terminal protein sequence, 2 other CAs, Soc and Joh (AJ), likely also derive from the kv325 gene [34]. While several of the KIII CAs are not identified by the anti-PSL3 reagent, sequence homologies and strong PSL2 reactivity suggest many (or all) may be kv325 derived. While the origin of certain of these KIII anti-I CAs is still uncertain, it is possible that they are kv325 derived but lack the

Table 3. IgM-KIII anti-I CAs [adapted from refs 49 and 62]

		Light chain			Heavy chain		
		anti-KIII subgroup	anti-PSL2	anti-PSL3	anti-subgroup I	anti-subgroup II	anti-subgroup III
1	Joh (AJ)*	+	+	–	–	+	–
2	Bat	+	+	+	–	+	–
3	Bon	+	+	–	–	+	–
4	Gag	NT	+	–	NT	NT	NT
5	Hig	+	+	–	–	+	–
6	Kau*	+	+	+	–	+	–
7	Lea	+	+	–	–	+	–
8	Per	+	+	–	–	+	–
9	Pos*	+	+	+	–	+	–
10	Soc*	+	+	–	–	+	–
11	Tri*	+	+	+	–	+	–

Compilation of serologic reactivities of antipeptide antisera with reduced and alkylated H and L chains by immunoblotting. All cold agglutinins bind I determinants on human erythrocytes. (*) designates that protein sequence analysis suggests that these L chains are kv325 derived [34; unpublished data]. Reactivity with anti-PSL3 is highly specific for kv325-derived L chains. The anti-subgroup II reagent is specific for VHIV gene encoded H chains.

PSL3 marker. Reactivity may have been lost due to: (1) somatic mutation causing critical residue substitutions, or (2) the effect of J regions or junctional diversity in the PSL3 region. Alternatively, it is possible that the L chains of some anti-I CAs may have derived from other V genes within the KIII subgroup.

Idiotypy and H Chain Usage

In the early 1970s shared serologic reactivity was reported among CAs against I and i determinants [20]. In explanation, while anti-I antibodies are generally kappa and anti-i are lambda, peptide mapping suggested that similar H chains may be used in these antibodies [43]. Isolated H chains from antibodies to I or i were later found to often share idiotypic determinants [44]. The structural basis of these cross-reacting determinants was unknown, and limited sequence data suggested that H chains with diverse amino termini might be employed in these antibodies [35]. However, to date there have been no reports of the complete H chain sequence of an anti-I CA.

To investigate H chain use in anti-I CAs, we developed a series of H chain subgroup-specific reagents, analogous to the kappa subgroup antisera already described [40]. When these studies were initiated, little was known about the organization of the human VH gene locus. H chains were assigned to three subgroups based on homologies within variable region frameworks [45]. DNA hybridization studies of genetic complexity suggested that within human H chain subgroups by gene number III>I>II.

Recently, several new VH gene families have been described [46–48]. However, like murine VH genes, based on framework homologies the six known human VH gene families can still be placed into three sets, which likely represent the genetic equivalent of the protein subgroups. The peptide sequences used to make reagents specific for subgroups I, II, and III, were taken from deduced amino acid sequences from VHI, VHIV and VHIII genes, respectively. Studies with first framework linked synthetic peptides have demonstrated that the subgroup I specific antibody may also have activity against the homologous portion of a protein derived from the newly described VHV gene, due to structural similarities with VHI-derived proteins [unpubl. observation]. Similarly, by ELISA the subgroup II specific reagent (derived from a VHIV gene sequence) reacts weakly with the VHII gene derived sequence, but is nonreactive with the other two protein subgroups (fig. 2). Recent studies suggest it is VHIV gene product specific. The diagnostic specificity of these antipeptide reagents has been confirmed by immunoblotting of VHI and VHIII H chains of known sequence (table 4).

When a collection of ten KIII anti-I CAs were studied (of which most are probably kv325 encoded), all were identified as using VHIV-derived H chains (fig. 3) [49]. Amino acid sequence data of H chains of this subgroup have rarely been reported, probably as most have a pyrrolidone carboxylic acid at the amino terminus that blocks sequential degradation. Significantly, this pattern of restricted H-L chain pairing in anti-I CAs is completely distinct from the VHI preference demonstrated in a collection of 30 KIIIb monoclonal rheumatoid factors (linked to the germline kv325 gene) [49]. This suggests that KIIIb L chains may possess multiple antigen-binding potentials. The binding specificity of antibodies with this L chain may therefore be defined by the H chains. This hypothesis is consistent with the finding that three KIIIb monoclonal antibodies to low density lipoprotein, and one KIIIb monoclonal antibody to intermediate filaments all use VHIII-encoded H chains [unpubl. observation]. Other support comes from the recent experiments

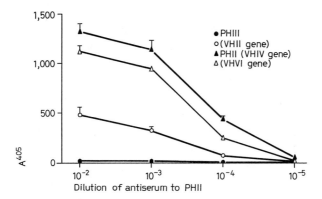

Fig. 2. Antipeptide reactivity of the VHII subgroup specific reagent. Antiserum was derived by immunization of a rabbit with the PHII synthetic peptide conjugated to keyhole limpet hemocyanin. The PHII peptide (△) represents a deduced sequence from a portion of the first framework sequence of the H chain of the 71-2 V gene, which has recently been assigned to the VHIV gene family [48]. Homologous sequences were used to make synthetic peptides specific for the VHIII (○) (from the CE1 V gene) and VHVI (△) (from the 15P1V gene) families, which are also VH subgroup II related [47, 63]. The four peptides were precoated at 2 μg/ml on separate microtiter wells, then nonspecific binding was later quenched with bovine serum albumin. Rabbit antiserum raised against PHII was then added at serial dilutions. After incubation and washing, binding of antiserum to each peptide was measured by enzyme linked immunoassay. The anti-PHII, subgroup II reagent, reacts differently with homologous peptides from the VHII, VHIV, and VHVI gene families (probably due to sequence homology), but not with the VHIII subgroup diagnostic peptide, PHIII (table 4). By immunoblot analysis anti-PHII is specific for VHIV gene products.

of Newkirk et al. [50], who reported that recombination of the kv325-derived L chain from EV1-15 (an antibody to cytomegalovirus) with the VHI H chain from Bor (an RF) created a hybrid with RF activity [50].

Discussion

Efforts in our laboratory have been directed at characterizing the H and L chains used in anti-I CAs. All anti-I antibodies use VHIV-derived H chains that primarily pair with L chains from a subset of VKIII genes. As stated above, the VH genes within the subgroup II may derive from at least three gene families. Of these families, VHIV may have seven or more germline genes, and VHII a smaller number of genes, but there is only one

Table 4. Specificity of human heavy chain subgroup reagents [adapted from ref. 41]

	Sequences of first framework peptides														Subgroup reactivity		
	9	10	11	12	13	14	15	16	17	18	19	20	21	22	anti subgroup I	anti subgroup II	anti subgroup III
VHI																	
PHI	A	E	V	K	K	P	G	A	S	V	K	V	S	C	–		–
Sie	–	–	–	–	–	–	–	S	–	–	R	–	T	–	+	–	–
Wol	–	–	–	–	–	–	–	S	–	–	R	–	–	–	+	–	–
Bor	–	–	–	–	–	–	–	S	–	–	–	–	T	–	+	–	–
Kas	–	–	–	–	–	–	–	S	–	–	–	–	–	–	+	–	–
VHIV																	
PHII	P	G	L	V	K	P	S	E	T	L	S	L	L	C	–	+	–
15P1	–	A	–	–	–	–	–	Q	–	–	–	–	–	–	–	+	–
CE1	–	A	–	–	–	A	T	H	T	–	T	–	–	–	–	+	–
VHIII																	
PHIII	G	G	L	V	Q	P	G	G	S	L	R	L	S	C	–	–	
Pom	–	–	–	–	–	–	–	–	–	–	–	–	–	–	–	–	+
Lay	–	–	–	–	–	–	–	–	–	–	–	–	–	–	–	–	+
Wea	–	–	–	–	E	–	S	–	–	–	–	–	–	–	–	–	+
Riv	–	–	V	–	–	–	–	–	–	–	–	–	–	–	–	–	+

Numbering according to Kabat et al. The synthetic peptides used to derive VH subgroups I, II, and III specific antisera are designated PHI, PHII, and PHIII, respectively. Except for Wea, all other IgMs were reported by Capra and co-workers. The sequence of the non-RF, Wea, was previously reported [45]. Reactivity of the paraprotein with the antiserum by immunoblotting is indicated by (+); lack of reactivity is indicated by (–). 15P1 and CE1 represent synthetic peptides derived from deduced sequences from prototype VHII and VHVI genes, respectively [48, 54, 62]. For these peptides reactivity was tested by immunoassay (fig. 2). Les was used as control for a VHIV-encoded H chain, based on DNA sequence analysis. By immunoblot analysis, the anti-subgroup II is specific for VHIV gene products. Adapted from Silverman et al. [40] and manuscript in preparation.

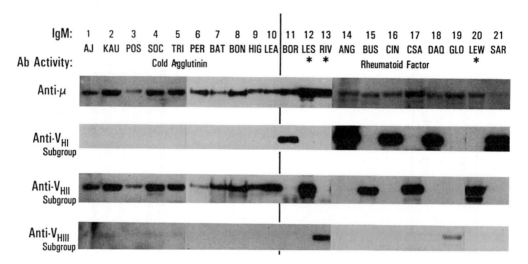

Fig. 3. Immunoblot analysis of the H chains of monoclonal IgM CAs and RFs. After SDS-PAGE separation and transfer to nitrocellulose, replicate blots of the H chains of ten IgM CAs and eleven IgM RFs were reacted with the indicated antipeptide antibodies. The anti-mu antiserum was derived with a sequence within the amino-terminal end of the mu constant region. (*) represents RFs which use non-KIIIb L chains based on sequence comparison. All other RFs use homologous KIIIb L chains likely derived from the kv325 germline gene. Most of the CAs bear serologic markers that suggest they are also kv325 derived. Of KIIIb autoantibodies, the CAs are restricted to VHII subgroup H chains encoded by VHIV genes, while the RFs display preferential pairing (5/8) with VHI H chains. Adapted from Silverman et al. [49].

VHVI gene. Significantly, the VHVI gene is probably the most J proximal [47]. For their relative number, subgroup II and KIII V genes are disproportionately used in lymphoid malignancies [51–53], and by paraproteins with autoimmune activity. Subgroup II H chains are often used in anti-I CAs and in kv328-derived monoclonal rheumatoid factors [manuscript in preparation]. However, based on idiotypic assays the subgroup II H chains used in KIIIa RFs appear distinct from those used in CAs [unpubl. observation].

Two processes could explain the prominence of subgroup II H chains in lymphoproliferative and autoimmune disorders. Either these genes are preferentially rearranged during certain stages of B cell development, or due to binding specificity B cells using these genes are stimulated to expand clonally, increasing their neoplastic potential. Evidence exists for both proposals. Certain genes of the VHIV family are rearranged preferentially during early development [54], and autoreactive B cells have been shown to represent a large part of the murine repertoire [55, 56]. Therefore, it is possible that both processes are contributory.

From our studies it is clear that VH and VL gene restriction within antibodies of anti-I specificity is the basis of the genetic and structural relatedness of these antibodies. However, anti-I CAs may express a variety of fine specificities. Further, severity of CA-associated clinical disease is correlated with both concentration and complement-fixing ability of the monoclonal CA, as well as reactivity at higher temperatures (or thermal amplitude) [23]. This latter property may be the result of somatic processes on these anticarbohydrate antibodies. Murine IgM antibodies to dextran have exhibited point mutations [57], and in one example an H chain residue substitution resulted in the addition of carbohydrate residues within a CDR and greater binding affinity [58]. Therefore, future efforts to assign structure-function correlates in anti-I CAs will require exact sequence determinations. Thereby the specific VHIV gene will be identified, and the contribution of J and D segments and somatic mutation to binding specificity can be assessed.

Summary

Cold agglutinins likely represent natural autoantibodies with precursors that arise early during ontogeny. Many use L chains derived from the germline kv325 gene, in association with H chains derived from the VHIV gene family. CAs probably represent an expression of the preimmune repertoire. The appearance of CAs in a variety of disorders may be due to the prevalence of CA B cell precursors, and the ubiquity of their target epitopes. CAs may arise independent of antigenic selection during Epstein-Barr virus infection in response to the expansion of immature B cells. In support, L chains bearing the markers for the kv325 gene are preferentially expressed during in vitro and in vivo Epstein-Barr virus infection [59]. Certain CAs that arise in lymphoproliferative disorders represent a clonal expansion, produced by karyotypically abnormal lymphocytes [60]. As such, antigenic selection may foster the early expansion of CA-producing clones. These cells are later more prone to become autonomous, and overt malignancy may then occur. Clues to the genetic origin of these antibodies are now being appreciated, but further study will be required to understand the defects responsible for the transformation of a natural autoantibody into a malignancy.

References

1   Duggan, D.B.; Schattner, A.: Unusual manifestations of monoclonal gammopathies. Am. J. Med. *81:* 864–870 (1986).

2   Hakomori, S.: Blood group ABH and Ii antigens of human erythrocytes. Chemistry, polymorphism, and their developmental change. Semin. Hematol. *18:* 39 (1981).

3   Fukuda, M.; Fukuda, M.N.; Papayannopoulou, T.; et al.: Membrane differentiation in human erythroid cells. Unique profiles of cell surface glycoproteins expressed in erythroblasts in vitro from three ontogenic stages. Proc. natn. Acad. Sci. USA *77:* 3474–3478 (1980).

4   Marcus, D.M.: A review of the immunogenic and immunomodulatory properties of glycosphingolipids. Mol. Immunol. *21:* 1083–1091 (1984).

5   Watanabe, K.; Laine, R.A.; Hakomori, S.-I.: On neutral fucoglycolipids having long, branched carbohydrate chains. H-active and I-active glycosphingolipids in human erythrocyte membranes. Biochem. J. *14:* 2725–2733 (1975).

6   Feizi, T.; Kabat, E.A.: Immunochemical studies on blood groups. J. exp. Med. *135:* 1247 (1972).

7   Adinolfi, M.: Anti-I antibody in normal newborn infants. Immunology *9:* 43–52 (1965).

8   Dube, V.E.; Tanaka, M.; Chmiel, J.; et al.: Effect of ABO group, secretor status and sex on cold hemmagglutinins in normal adults. Vox Sang. *46:* 75–79 (1984).

9   Pennington, J.; Feizi, T.: Horse anti-type XIV pneumococcus sera behave as cold agglutinins recognizing developmentally regulated antigens apart from the Ii antigens on human erythrocytes. Vox Sang. *43:* 253–258 (1982).

10 Lefrançois, G.; Le Bras, J.; Bouvet, E.; et al.: Anti-erythrocyte autoimmunisation during chronic falciparum malaria. Lancet *1981:* 661–663.

11 Duran-Suarez, J.R.; Martin-Vega, C.; Argelagues, E.; et al.: Red cell I antigen as immune complex receptor in drug-induced hemolytic anemias. Vox Sang. *41:* 313–315 (1981).

12 Murray, W.H.; Masur, H.; Senterfit, L.B.; et al.: The protean manifestations of *Mycoplasma pneumoniae* infection in adults. Am. J. Med. *58:* 229 (1988).

13 Feizi, T.; Schumacher, M.: Light chain homogeneity of post-infective cold agglutinins. Clin. exp. Immunol. *3:* 923–929 (1968).

14 Feizi, T.: Lambda chains in cold agglutinins. Science *156:* 1111–1112 (1987).

15 Feizi, T.; Taylor-Robinson, D.; Shields, M.D.; et al.: Production of cold agglutinins in rabbits immunized with human erythrocytes treated with *Mycoplasma pneumoniae*. Nature, Lond. *222:* 1253–1256 (1969).

15a Loomes, L.M.; Uemura, K.; Childs, R.A.; et al.: Erythrocyte receptors for *Mycoplasma pneumoniae* are sialylated oligosaccharide of Ii antigen type. Nature, Lond. *307:* 560–563 (1984).

16 Pruzanski, W.; Cowan, D.H.; Parr, D.M.: Clinical and immunochemical studies of IgM cold agglutinins with lambda type light chains. Clin. Immunol. Immunopathol. *2:* 234–245 (1974).

17 Roelcke, D.; Ebert, W.; Feizi, T.: Studies on the specificities of two IgM lambda cold agglutinins. Immunology *27:* 879–886 (1974).

18 Capra, J.D.; Dowling, P.; Cook, S.; et al.: An incomplete cold-reactive gamma G antibody with i specificity in infectious mononucleosis. Vox Sang. *16:* 10–17 (1969).

19 Freedman, J.; Newland, M.: Autoimmune haemolytic anaemia with the unusual combination of both IgM and IgG autoantibodies. Vox Sang. *32:* 61–68 (1977).

20 Lecomte, J.; Feizi, T.: A common idiotype on human macroglobulins with anti-I and anti-i specificity. Clin. exp, Immunol. *20:* 287–302 (1975).

21 Roelcke, D.; Anstee, D.J.; Jungfer, H.; et al.: IgG-type cold agglutinins in children and corresponding antigens. Vox Sang. *20:* 218–229 (1971).

22 Marcus, D.M.; Kundu, S.K.; Suzuki, A.: The P blood group system. Recent progress in immunochemistry and genetics. Semin. Hematol. *18:* 63 (1981).

23 Pruzanski, W.; Shumak, K.H.: Biologic activity of cold-reacting autoantibodies. New Engl. J. Med. *297:* 538–542 (1977).

24 Riesen, W.F.; Majaniemi, I.; Huser, H.; et al.: Variable-region subgroup and specificity of cold agglutinins. Scand. J. Immunol. *8:* 145–148 (1978).

25 Wang, A.C.: A new subgroup of the kappa chain variable region associated with anti-Pr cold agglutinin. Nature New Biol. *243:* 126 (1973).

26 Lorenz, W.; Schable, K.F.; Thiebe, R.; et al.: The J kappa ·proximal region of the human K locus contains three uncommon V kappa genes which are arranged in opposite transcriptional polarities. Mol. Immunol. *215:* 479–484 (1988).

27 Yancopoulos, G.D.; Desiderio, S.V.; Paskind, M.; et al.: Preferential utilization of the most JH-proximal VH gene segments in pre-B-cell lines. Nature *311:* 727–731 (1984).

28 Klobeck, H.-G.; Bornkamm, G.W.; Combriato, G.; et al.: Subgroup IV of human immunoglobulin K light chains is encoded by a single germline gene. Nucl. Acids Res. *13:* 6515–6528 (1985).

29 Feizi, T.; Kunkel, H.G.; Roelcke, D.: Cross idiotypic specificity among cold agglutinins in relation to combining activity for blood group-related antigens. Clin. exp. Immunol. *18:* 283–293 (1974).

30 Capra, J.D.; Kehoe, J.M.: Variable region sequences of five human immunoglobulin heavy chains of the V_HIII subgroup. Definite identification of four heavy chain hypervariable regions. Proc. natn. Acad. Sci. USA *71:* 845–848 (1974).

31 Williams, R.C., Jr.; Kunkel, H.G.; Capra, J.D.: Antigenic specificities related to the cold agglutinin activity of gamma M globulins. Science *161:* 379–381 (1968).

32 Harboe, M.; Van Furth, R.; Schubothe, H.; et al.: Exclusive occurrence of K chains in isolated cold hemagglutinins. Scand. J. Haematol. *2:* 259–266 (1965).

33 Feizi, T.; Lecomte, J.; Childs, R.; et al.: Kappa chain (V kappa III) subgroup-related activity in an idiotypic anti-cold agglutinin serum. Scand. J. Immunol. *5:* 629–636 (1976).

34 Capra, J.D.; Kehoe, J.M.; Williams, R.C., Jr.; et al.: Light chain sequences of human IgM cold agglutinins. Proc. natn. Acad. Sci. USA *69:* 40 (1972).

35 Gergely, J.; Wang, A.C.; Fudenberg, H.H.: Chemical analyses of variable regions of heavy and light chains of cold agglutinins. Vox Sang. *24:* 432–440 (1970).

36 Chen, P.P.; Albrandt, K.; Kipps, T.J.; et al.: Isolation and characterization of human VkIII germline genes. Implications for the molecular basis of human VkIII light chain diversity. J. Immun. *139:* 1727–1733 (1987).

37 Pons-Estel, B.; Goni, F.; Solomon, A.; et al.: Sequence similarities among kIIIb chains of monoclonal human IgMk autoantibodies. J. exp. Med. *160:* 893–904 (1984).

38 Chen, P.P.; Fong, S.; Normansell, D.; et al.: Delineation of a cross-reactive idiotype on human autoantibodies with antibody against a synthetic peptide. J. exp. Med. *159:* 1502–1511 (1984).

39 Silverman, G.J.; Carson, D.A.; Solomon, A.; et al.: Human kappa light chain subgroup analysis with synthetic peptide-induced antisera. J. immunol. Methods *95:* 249–257 (1986).

40 Silverman, G.J.; Goldfien, R.D.; Chen, P.; et al.: Idiotypic and subgroup analysis of human monoclonal rheumatoid factors. Implications for structural and genetic basis of autoantibodies in humans. J. clin. Invest. *82:* 469–475 (1988).

41 Chen, P.P.; Robbins, D.L.; Jirik, F.R.; et al.: Isolation and characterization of a light chain variable region gene for human rheumatoid factors. J. exp. Med. *166:* 1900–1905 (1987).

42 Newkirk, M.M.; Capra, J.D.: Cross-idiotypic specificity among human rheumatoid factors. Monogr. Allergy *22:* 1–11 (1987).

43 Cooper, A.G.; Chavin, S.I.; Franklin, E.C.: Predominance of a single mu chain subclass in cold agglutinin heavy chains. Immunochemistry *7:* 479–483 (1970).

44 Childs, R.; Feizi, T.: Cross idiotypic specificity among heavy chains of macroglobulins with blood group I and i specificities. Nature, Lond. *255:* 562–564 (1975).

45 Kabat, E.A.; Wu, T.T.; Reid-Miller, M.; et al.: Sequences of proteins of immunological interest. (US Department of Health & Human Services, Washington 1987).

46 Humphries, C.G.; Shen, A.; Kuziel, W.A.; et al.: A new human immunoglobulin V_H family preferentially rearranged in immature B-cell tumours. Nature, Lond. *331:* 446–449 (1988).

47 Berman, J.E.; Mellis, S.J.; Pollock, R.; et al.: Content and organization of the human Ig VH locus. Definition of three new VH families and linkage to the Ig CH locus. Eur. molec. biol. Org. J.*7:* 727–738 (1988).

48 Lee, K.H.; Matsuda, F.; Kinashi, T.; et al.: A novel family of variable region genes of the human immunoglobulin heavy chain. J. molec. Biol. *195:* 761–768 (1987).

49 Silverman, G.J.; Goni, F.; Chen, P.P.; et al.: Distinct patterns of heavy chain variable region subgroup use by human monoclonal autoantibodies of different specificity. J. exp. Med. *168:* 2361–2366 (1988).

50 Newkirk, M.M.; Gram, H.; Heinrich, G.F.; et al.: The complete protein sequences of the variable regions of the cloned heavy and light chains of a human anti-cytomegalovirus antibody reveal a striking similarity to human rheumatoid factors of the Wa idiotypic family. J. clin. Invest. *81:* 1151 (1988).

51 Bird, J.; Galili, N.; Link, M.; et al.: Continuing rearrangement but absence of somatic hypermutation in immunoglobulin genes of human B cell precursor leukemia. J. exp. Med. *168:* 229–245 (1988).

52 Kipps, T.J.; Robbins, B.A.; Kuster, P.; et al.: Autoantibody-associated cross-reactive idiotypes expressed at high frequency in chronic lymphocytic leukemia relative to B-cell lymphomas of follicular center cell origin. Blood *72:* 422–428 (1988).

53 Silverman, G.J.; Fong, S.; Chen, P.P.; et al.: Clinical update: Cross reactive idiotypes and the genetic origin of rheumatoid factors. J. clin. Lab. Analyt. *1:* 129–135 (1987).

54 Schroeder, H.W., Jr.; Hillman, J.L.; Perlmutter, R.M.: Early restriction of the human antibody repertoire. Science *238:* 791–793 (1987).

55 Painter, C.; Monestier, M.; Bonin, B.; et al.: Functional and molecular studies of V genes expressed in autoantibodies. Immunol. Rev. *94:* 75–98 (1986).

56 Portnoi, D.; Freitas, A.; Holmberg, D.; et al.: Immunocompetent autoreactive B lymphocytes are activated cycling cells in normal mice. J. exp. Med. *164:* 25–35 (1986).

57 Hartman, A.B.; Rudikoff, S.: V_H genes encoding the immune response to beta-(1,6)-galactan: Somatic mutation in IgM molecules. Eur. molec. biol. Org. J. *3:* 3023–3030 (1984).

58 Wallick, S.C.; Kabat, E.A.; Morrison, S.L.: Glycosylation of a V_H residue of a monoclonal antibody against alpha(1>6) dextran increases its affinity for antigen. J. exp. Med. *168:* 1099–1109 (1988).

59 Silverman, G.J.; Carson, D.A.; Patrick, K.; et al.: Expression of a germline human kappa chain associated cross reactive idiotype after in vitro and in vivo infection with Epstein-Barr virus. Clin. Immunol. Immunopathol. *43:* 403–411 (1987).

60 Silberstein, L.E.; Robertson, G.A.; Harris, A.C.H.; et al.: Etiologic aspects of cold agglutinin disease. Evidence for cytogenetically defined clones of lymphoid cells and the demonstration that an anti-Pr cold autoantibody is derived from a chromosomally aberrant B cell clone. Blood *67:* 1705–1709 (1988).

61 Edman, P.; Cooper, A.G.: Amino acid sequence at the N-terminal end of a cold agglutinin kappa chain. FEBS Lett. *2:* 33–35 (1968).

62 Agnello, V.; Goni, F.; Barnes, J.L.; et al.: Human rheumatoid factor crossidiotypes. II. Primary structure-dependent crossreactive idiotype, PSL2-CRI, present on Wa monoclonal rheumatoid factors is present on B1a and other IgMk monoclonal autoantibodies. J. exp. Med. *165:* 263–267 (1987).

63 Kodaira, M.; Kinashi, T.; Umemura, I.; et al.: Organization and evolution of variable region genes of the human immunoglobulin heavy chain. J. molec. Biol. *190:* 529–541 (1986).

Gregg J. Silverman, MD, Department of Basic and Clinical Research (BCR4),
10666 North Torrey Pines Road, La Jolla, CA 92037 (USA)

Carson DA, Chen PP, Kipps TJ (eds): Idiotypes in Biology and Medicine.
Chem Immunol. Basel, Karger, 1990, vol 48, pp 126–166

Anti-Idiotypic Therapy of Leukemias and Lymphomas

Freda K. Stevenson, Andrew J.T. George, Martin J. Glennie

Lymphoma Research Unit, Tenovus Research Laboratory, General Hospital,
Southampton, UK

Introduction

The idea of specific attack on tumor cells, either by the use of passive
monoclonal antibody or by active immunization, requires that the target cell
should display a tumor-associated antigen (TAA). Generally, such antigens
have been difficult to detect and define chemically until the advent of a range
of monoclonal antibodies and the techniques of molecular biology. However,
for the majority of B cell tumors, both human and animal, the idiotypic
determinants of the surface immunoglobulin (Ig) carried by the tumor cells
represent well-defined TAAs. Surface Ig, while capable of acting as a TAA, is
also a molecule with a known function in the normal immune response,
which might itself be subject to control by regulatory anti-idiotypic pathways
[1]. Clearly, when a B cell tumor develops, the host's putative anti-idiotypic
control has failed. Restoration of such control might occur after the reduction in tumor load which can occur after antibody therapy [2, 3]. Expansion
of anti-idiotypic pathways might be encouraged by immunizing the host with
tumor-derived idiotypic Ig. This is an attractive concept since, once in place,
it should act against emerging tumor cells on a continuing basis.

An ideal approach to therapy could combine both passive and active
treatments whereby tumor load is reduced with anti-idiotypic antibody, with
no significant deleterious effects on the ability of the host to mount an
immune response. This would allow a subsequent active immunization with
idiotypic Ig. This active immunization could also be given to patients who

have not been treated with antibody but who have responded to a mild course of chemotherapy. If a relatively stable remission has been induced, the damage to the patient's normal cells by the chemotherapy may be minimal or at least recoverable before tumor reappears. In this case there would be a time period where immunization could be contemplated.

Both passive and active immunotherapeutic approaches require that the target cells continue to express the idiotypic determinants at the cell surface and, although clinical benefit should still be seen, the considerable ability of target cells to avoid immune attack might well lead to emergence of tumor variants. Passive antibody treatment with monoclonal anti-idiotypic antibody has revealed the loss of expression of idiotypic determinants at the cell surface by both temporary [4] and more permanent [5] mechanisms. Temporary antigenic modulation can be dealt with to some extent by the use of univalent antibodies [6], either simple FabFc combinations or as bispecific antibodies where the second antibody can bind either a toxin or an effector cell [7]. These kinds of derivatives appear more effective than simple unmodified bivalent monoclonal antibodies which have proved rather disappointing [8]. More permanent loss of an idiotope at the cell surface can occur after therapy [5] and this will require attack at more than one idiotope. Total loss of Ig expression as a result of antibody therapy has not yet been observed for human lymphoma, although it has been found in a number of animal leukemias following treatment with various reagents including immunotoxins [9]. Clearly, this would prevent further use of the idiotypic determinants as TAA.

Problems in the use of active immunization with idiotypic Ig arise at two major points: first, in the establishment of an anti-idiotypic immune response in a patient who might have some degree of immunosuppression due either to tumor or to previous chemotherapy. There is a theoretical possibility that specific tolerance to the idiotypic Ig might exist in the patient: this is a question which needs investigation. The second point where problems could arise overlaps with the tumor escape mechanisms mentioned earlier. The situation is slightly different, however, since active immunization must generate a polyclonal host response against all available idiotopes, leading to emergence of only Ig-negative variants. This has been demonstrated for a mouse lymphoma [10]. However, such a consequence may not prove to be a disaster, since the two surface Ig-negative variants which did eventually emerge from anti-idiotypic restraint both showed a slower growth rate than the original tumor, leading to the suggestion that the presence of Ig at the cell surface might affect division rate in B cell tumors. Clearly, there is a great deal to be learned about the behavior of tumor cells under immune pressure, some of which will have implications for immunotherapy of other forms of cancer. The present review attempts to assess the current status of both the passive and active approaches to immunotherapy of B cell tumors.

Novel Antibodies in the Treatment of Lymphoma

Although the impact of monoclonal antibodies in the treatment of human neoplastic disease has been less than might have been hoped, some useful and encouraging results have been obtained. This is particularly true for B cell lymphomas treated with anti-idiotype antibodies [11]. While the need for anti-idiotype antibodies to be tailor-made for each patient is an undoubted drawback to this approach, their specificity has been a major boon, particularly before the days of monoclonal technology. The general poor level of response to treatment has not been due to any lack of antibody: in some cases patients have relapsed or failed to respond despite cumulative doses greater than 3 g of anti-idiotype. The usual result following treatment with antibody alone is a partial and transient diminution of tumor load, manifesting as a rapid but short-lived removal of any circulating tumor cells with, in perhaps 50% of cases, significant reductions in solid deposits following prolonged treatment [8]. By far the most successful result was achieved in the first patient to be given monoclonal anti-idiotype [3]. Here the patient remained apparently tumor-free for some 6 years before eventually relapsing with the original tumor (reactive with the anti-idiotype used in treatment).

While such results have been disappointing therapeutically, there have been positive aspects to this work, in particular the identification of a number of factors able to thwart antibody treatment [11]. Prominent among these factors is the process of antigenic modulation in which antibody-coated cells first redistribute and then clear the surface antibody-antigen complexes, providing them with a temporary but effective means of escape from immune attack [4, 6, 12]. Surface Ig is particularly susceptible to antigenic modulation, offering tumor a route of escape from both passive and active immunotherapy (see below). These studies have also shown that tumors, because of their heterogeneous nature, always have the potential to escape attack from any single antibody through mutational loss of surface antigen [5, 9], and thus present a case in favor of attacking tumors with more than one antibody. Another important factor in reducing antibody efficacy has been the blocking of antibody access to the tumor cell surface, either by extracellular antigen in the form of secreted Ig idiotype or by anti-rodent Ig antibody response in the patient. The problem of anti-Ig responses has been less severe in B lymphoid neoplasia than in other tumors, presumably reflecting their often severe level of immunosuppression, but nevertheless even in these tumors it has some-times required the antibody treatment to be stopped [8].

Finally, there is the whole question of which effectors are most appropri-ate in tumor therapy, the level at which such effectors exist in tumor patients and which antibodies are most suitable to harness them. While it is clear that some rodent antibodies will be better than others [13], rat IgG2b appearing particularly effective, most lack potency with human effectors especially for recruiting complement and are unlikely to harness the full potential of the human immune system. The action of anti-idiotype antibodies alone has not been observed to compromise the viability of tumor cells. Evidence from animal studies [11, 14] and in vitro investigations [15] suggest that the therapeutic effects which have been recorded in patients result from recruit-ment of cellular effectors, with the monocyte [16, 17] and the large granular lymphocyte [15, 18], being leading contenders as mediators of such effects. However, with the appropriate antibody or antibody derivative it may be possible to recruit these and other, more potent, effectors which until now have remained untapped.

Engineering More Effective Antibodies

In this section of the review we will consider some novel antibody derivatives currently being investigated for attacking neoplastic targets including B cell lymphomas. They are designed to use two strategies for eliminating neoplastic cells: first, the recruitment of natural effectors such as cytotoxic cells of the immune system, and second the delivery of cytotoxic compounds such as a toxin to neoplastic cells, i.e. employing Paul Ehrlich's original concept of the specific antibody as a carrier molecule for highly toxic reagents [19, 20].

'Humanized' Antibodies

In an attempt to overcome at least two of the major limitations of rodent antibodies, their immunogenicity and lack of potency, a number of groups have embarked on programs to 'humanize' selected rodent antibodies. By this we mean the construction, by chemical synthesis or recombinant DNA technology, of derivatives in which rodent antibody-binding sites are stitched onto human Ig constant regions.

Our original work on humanizing rodent antibodies started back in the early 1980s [21]. We showed that functional antibodies could be generated by chemically coupling the Fab' fragment from a mouse anti-idiotype antibody onto intact human IgG or onto its Fc fragments via tandem thioether bonds. The synthesis was precise, in that it used a dimaleimide cross-linker to ensure that mainly hinge region SH groups were used in the coupling process, and was followed by exclusion chromatography to isolate just the required FabIgG or FabFc derivatives. The efficiency of the synthesis (about 40% in terms of starting Fab' antibody) meant that gram quantities of clinical grade material could be produced. Furthermore, because the derivatives carried human Fc regions, we were ensuring minimal immunogenicity, an extended biological survival and hopefully maximum therapeutic potency.

In addition to any advantage gained from presenting a patient's immune system with homologous Fc, we had anticipated that these derivatives, being univalent, should avoid the problem of antigenic modulation. Our previous work with the univalent antibody fragment, Fab/c, in which one Fab arm of a rabbit IgG antibody was removed by limited proteolysis with papain, had shown that in vitro at least, antibodies which bind via one arm fail to cross-link surface Ig, and are not removed from the cell surface by antigenic modulation [6]. We now know that univalent derivatives, including FabIgG and FabFc, despite being unable to cross-link surface antigen on the tumor cells, can still mediate a slow form of antigenic modulation in patients [22]. Work from Schroff's laboratory [23] and our own [22] has shown that in vivo antigenic modulation is probably enhanced or induced when FcR-bearing accessory cells, such as monocytes and Kupffer cells, cross-link antibody-antigen complexes on target cells. Thus, the therapeutic superiority of univalent antibody might simply reflect the fact that it does not induce the very rapid modulation which surface Ig normally exhibits [24].

The first patient to be treated with the FabIgG derivative of anti-idiotype was a 52-year-old woman with widespread B cell lymphoma of the nodular, centrocytic/centroblastic type, and with neoplastic cells present in the blood at about $7 \times 10^9/l$ [25]. A course of four infusions of 380–580 mg FabIgG was given over a period of 11 weeks. Each infusion was followed by a fall in the number of circulating neoplastic cells, reaching a minimum of 5–50% of the preinfusion level after about 24 h and then rising slowly over a period of about 10 days towards the original level. Four days after completion of each infusion, lymph nodes in all areas had swollen to about twice their previous size and were tender. They remained enlarged for 5–8 days and then subsided. Four weeks after completing the course of infusions, the number of circulating neoplastic cells was at about 50% of the pretreatment level, and the tumor masses were considered to have shrunk by rather more than 50%. The patient has remained well for over 2 years, with tumor masses unchanged and hemoglobin and granulocyte levels well maintained. Remarkably, the lymphocyte count continued to fall for some time after treatment had ceased. Thus, this patient underwent a partial remission in response to chimeric anti-idiotype, and then, in the unpredictable way of well-differentiated lymphomas, maintained a stationary tumor load throughout the ensuing period of observation.

Other B cell lymphoma patients are now receiving chimeric FabFc (now the derivative of choice for patient therapy), and preliminary results suggest they will show similar responses to that described for the first patient. The anticipated increase in metabolic survival of chimeric antibodies has now been confirmed. Control FabIgG without antibody activity for a patient's tumor, had a plasma half-life of >10 days, considerably longer than the <24 h reported for circulating mouse antibodies [26]. Furthermore, throughout these investigations we have seen no indications of any immune response to the infused antibody.

Recently we have described a new chimeric antibody, bisFabFc, for therapeutic use in man (fig. 1) [27]. This derivative is constructed when two FabFc molecules are linked together using a bismaleimide reagent to give an antibody with two Fc regions. As regards its antibody activity against target cells the bisFabFc can be univalent, bivalent, or bispecific. Its juxtaposed dual Fc regions are designed to promote cooperative binding of effectors, and already various bisFabFc have proved notably more powerful than the parent FabFc molecules in promoting complement lysis and ADCC. Distinguishing the relative contributions of Fc architecture, antibody affinity and other factors to this improvement in performance will be a long task. It appears that the bispecific bisFabFc molecules offer particular promise, since, in addition to having dual Fc regions for effector recruitment, its ability to recognize two distinct surface antigens should yield a higher affinity than shown by univalent derivatives, and reduce the chance of a variant antigen-negative cell escaping attack. What penalty in terms of enhanced antigenic modulation we must pay for these advantages is not known. Perhaps by selecting anti-idiotype along with one of the B cell-associated antigens, e.g. CD19 or CD37, which are not inclined to modulate,

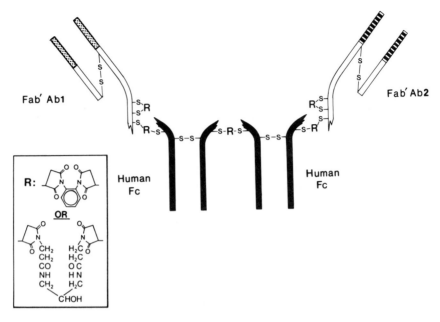

Fig. 1. Schematic diagram of a novel antibody, bisFabFc, designed for the efficient recruitment of effectors against neoplastic targets [27]. Three stages are involved in its construction: (1) antibody Fab′ fragments and human Fc fragments are prepared by pepsin and papain digestion of monoclonal antitarget cell antibody and normal human IgG, respectively; (2) univalent FabFc derivatives are prepared by linking Fab and Fc via hinge-region SH groups [25], and (3) pairs of FabFc molecules are linked together via a free SH group on the Fc as shown. The FabFc derivatives can be paired in various combinations, allowing the construction of bisFabFc molecules which are univalent, bivalent or bispecific (the figure represents a bispecific derivative). The juxtaposed dual Fc regions are designed to promote cooperative binding of effectors, and already various bisFabFc have proved notably more powerful than the parent FabFc molecules in promoting complement lysis and ADCC. The inset shows the linking groups (R) derived from the bismaleimide reagents, N,N′-o-phenylenedimaleimide (upper) and N,N′-bis(3-maleimidopropionyl)-2-hydroxy-1,3-propanediamine (lower). The former is preferred for the Fab′-Fc link, the latter for the inter-Fc link.

we can construct bispecific derivatives which remain comparatively specific for individual B cell tumors, but do not undergo rapid modulation.

Most workers in this field have chosen an alternative path to producing humanized antibodies, that is using recombinant DNA methodology [28–30]. The first step in this venture was to find suitable expression systems into which the modified Ig genes could be transfected. To date only mammalian B lymphoid cells which possess the appropriate Ig regulatory elements have proved suitable, with the mouse myeloma cell proving by far to be the most successful. Initial experiments demonstrated that it was possible to transfect myelomas and hybridomas, and that the introduced genes were expressed successfully in good quantity [28, 29]. Prokaryotic cells, while useful for expression of some interesting Ig fragments such as the Fv regions [31], have generally not been useful for production of intact antibodies.

Morrison et al. [29] reported in 1984 that by the appropriate manipulations of Ig exons it was possible to join the variable domains from a mouse antibody to the human constant region domains, thus generating an antibody which was mainly human. The integrity of such chimeric antibodies was such that antigen-binding and effector functions remained intact. Many antibodies have now been humanized in this way, including at least three examples in which all four of the human IgG isotypes have been linked to one set of rodent antibody-V regions [30, 32, 33]. Such matched series include the antileukocyte antibody, Campath-1, reactive with most lymphocytes and monocytes and used in the treatment of B cell malignancies [13, 30], plus the anti-adenocarcinoma antibody, 17-1A [26, 33]. In addition, Bruggemann et al. [32] have constructed a matched series of human antibodies specific for the hapten 4-hydroxy-3-nitrophenacetyl (NP), including the four IgG isotypes plus IgM, IgE and IgA2 antibodies. Humanized antibodies of this type have proved powerful reagents in analyzing the role of Ig isotype in the recruitment of natural effectors such as complement and cellular effectors. The IgG1 antibodies stand out as the most effective isotype, able to mediate effective target-cell lysis with both human peripheral blood mononuclear cells and human complement. The IgG3 isotype is the next most active antibody, with IgG2 and IgG4 proving relatively inactive. The efficiency of IgG1 antibody at activating human complement to lysis has been something of a surprise in view of the known superior performance of the IgG3 isotype at binding the first component of the complement cascade, C1q. Recently, Bindon et al. [34] have extended this work with a matched series of humanized antibodies binding to NIP-haptenized human red cells and measured the relative efficiency of IgG1 and IgG3 antibodies at each step in the complement cascade up to C3b binding. This work showed that while IgG3 antibody bound C1 more efficiently, that C1 bound by the IgG1 antibody was 10 times more efficient at delivering C4b and C3b molecules to the target membranes. This increased efficiency did not appear to arise through C4 molecules binding to the IgG1 antibody itself, and could simply reflect a relative inefficiency on the part of IgG3 due to its unusually long hinge leaving short-lived activated complement components some distance from the target membrane [35].

Recently, using similar genetic engineering, it has been possible to further refine humanized antibodies by genetically replacing just the six complementarity-determining (hypervariable) regions (three heavy and three light chains) of human IgG1 with those from the rat monoclonal Campath-1 [30]. This reshaped human antibody binds antigen, is as active as the parent rat IgG2b antibody in cytolysis with human complement, and is more active with human cellular effectors. Next to human antibodies they offer the best opportunity of exploiting the full potency of the human effector systems, while avoiding anti-antibody responses in the patient. There still remains the potential as with any monoclonal antibody, even human, of generating an anti-idiotype response. However, it seems likely that reshaped antibodies will allow extended periods of treatment before such responses become evident.

At the time of writing, results from immunotherapy studies with genetically engineered antibodies are not available. However, preliminary immunogenicity studies with the humanized anti-adenocarcinoma antibody, Ch-17-1A, in patients with metastatic colon carcinoma have been encouraging [39]. First, the chimeric antibody shows an extended half-life, remaining in the circulation of patients 4–10 times as long as the parent mouse antibody (17-1A). This is still shorter than the recorded half-life of IgG1 (21 days) [40] and shorter than the > 10 days reported by Hamblin et al. [25] (see above) for a chimeric FabIgG derivative comprising mouse Fab′ linked to human IgG. Second, pharmacokinetic studies in 10 patients with Ch-17-1A antibody showed that over a 12-week period only 1 patient developed an anti-idiotype response to the xenogeneic variable regions, this despite multiple infusions of up to three of 40 mg given at 2-week intervals [39]. The lack of any anti-idiotype response in the 9 other patients suggests that removing the major immunogenic portion of the protein not only circumvents the anti-isotype response, but also reduces the anti-idiotype component of the immune response [41]. Hopefully with human antibodies which have been reshaped with just rodent-derived hypervariable loops, immunogenicity will be reduced to a point where all patients, regardless of their immune status, can receive multiple treatments over extended periods.

While genetically mixing Ig exons provides a useful means of generating antibodies which should perform well in patients, the process of site-directed mutagenesis provides an opportunity of making more minor changes within Ig exons. Making these minor changes could allow us to identify precisely the site at which effector molecules bind to antibodies, and also to engineer novel humanized antibodies that utilize selected functions. Advances have already been made using this technology. First, Duncan et al. [36, 37] have 'pin-pointed' the binding site on human IgG for the macrophage high-affinity Fc receptor, FcRI, to the lower hinge region. They showed that by changing a single amino acid (residue 235) from Leu to Glu, IgG3 FcRI-binding activity was abolished. In contrast, in a reverse experiment using mouse IgG2b, which does not bind to FcRI, changing Glu 235 to Leu established such binding. Second, similar studies by Duncan and Winter [38] have located the binding site for C1q on human IgG to residues Glu 318, Lys 320 and Lys 322 of the C_H2. Even with just these two binding sites identified we are in a position to consider engineering antibodies with novel activity, for example, to construct human antibodies which retain activity with complement but no longer bind to FcR on cells of the reticuloendothelial system. As more receptor-binding sites are located, so we should gain increased control over which effector functions are recruited.

Bispecific Antibodies

One of the latest developments in novel antitumor agents is the bispecific Ab. These are reagents with dual specificity for antigen which can be used as highly selective and adaptable heterobifunctional cross-linkers. For example, in immunocytochemistry and immunoassays they can couple a selected antigen to a detecting agent such as ferritin or horseradish peroxidase in a single step, doing away with the need for covalently coupled immunoconjugates [42–44]. Milstein and colleagues [45] have shown that they appear to have particular advantages for staining of tissue sections, giving improvements in sensitivity, signal-to-noise ratios, and an unusually uniform staining pattern across entire tissue sections. More recently, we have also shown that bispecific antibody of the appropriate specificity can be used to link a fluorochrome such as phycoerythrin to target cells and allow immunofluorescence analysis by FACS [7]. While such applications may be useful, far greater interest lies in their potential as therapeutic agents [7, 46–53]. Unwanted cells, including neoplastic and virally infected cells, have been attacked in two ways: first using bispecific antibody designed to recruit cellular effectors [45–49], such as CTL and large granular lymphocytes (LGL); and, second, with bispecific antibody capable of linking cytotoxic agents such as drugs and toxins to target cells [7, 50–52].

Until recently three types of bispecific derivative have been prominent in the literature (fig. 2). The first of these, bispecific F(ab')$_2$, was prepared as

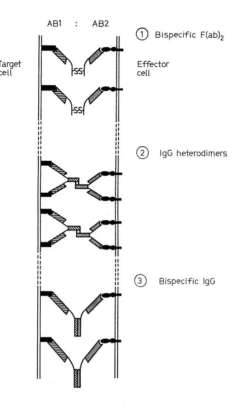

Fig. 2. Three types of bispecific antibody in current use for the recruitment of cellular effectors and the targeting of cytotoxic agents. (1) Bispecific F(ab')$_2$ antibody formed by the oxidation of hinge-region SH groups of two antibody Fab'$_{SH}$ fragments [42]. (2) Bispecific IgG heterodimers formed when two monoclonal IgG antibodies are coupled by a chemical cross-linker such as SPDP [46, 47]. (3) Bispecific IgG secreted as one of the Ig products of a hybrid-hybridoma [44, 45].

early as 1962, when Nisonoff and Mandy [43] demonstrated that reduced Fab' fragments from two rabbit antibodies could be re-oxidized via their hinge-region SH groups to form F(ab')$_2$ heterodimers, a proportion of which showed bispecific activity. More recently this approach has been modified and by directed disulfide exchange it is now possible to generate pure heterodimer populations using any pair of antibody Fab' fragments [54].

With the advent of monoclonal technology two other approaches have been employed to provide bispecific derivatives. The more straightforward involves the production of 'heteroaggregates' or 'heterodimers' of IgG in

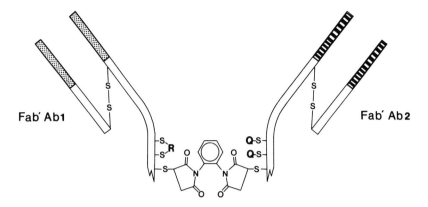

Fig. 3. Bispecific F(ab')₂ antibody containing Fab' fragments (Fab' Ab1 and Fab' Ab2) from two mouse IgG1 antibodies. Groups joined to cysteinyl sulfur: Q = carboxyamidomethyl; R = *o*-phenylenedisuccimimidyl (as depicted linking the two Fd chains via thioether bonds).

which two monoclonal antibodies are simply joined using a lysine-reactive/SH-reactive cross-linker such as N-succinimidyl-3(2-pyridyldithiol) propionate (SPDP) [46, 47]. The various products can then be fractionated by chromatography to obtain polymers of the required size. A more complex but ultimately more promising approach involves the construction by cell fusion of hybrid hybridomas which secrete the products of two Ab-producing cells [44, 45]. The four Ig polypeptide chains, two heavy and two light, will be codominantly expressed and can associate to form a mixture of hybrid IgG molecules, a proportion of which will express both antibody specificities. Fortunately, the various H-L combinations are usually not randomly expressed, and preferential association between homologous H and L chains to form functional binding sites can result in 20% of the Ig being bispecific. Nevertheless, isolating this material remains difficult. While conventional chromatography sometimes gives a partial resolution of the hybrid molecules it will probably require techniques such as isoelectric focusing or chromatofocusing to yield anything like pure bispecific Ab.

Recently we have developed a fourth type of bispecific F(ab')₂ antibody in which pairs of Fab' fragments are linked together via their hinge region SH groups, using a thioether linkage [7] (fig. 3). Briefly, peptic F(ab')₂ fragments from the two chosen antibodies are first reduced to provide Fab'$_{SH}$. The SH groups on one of the Fab'$_{SH}$ partners are then fully alkylated with o-phenylenedimaleimide (o-PDM) to provide free maleimide groups. Finally, the two preparations, Fab'_{mal} and Fab'_{SH}, are combined under conditions which allow cross-linking of the maleimide and SH groups and avoid re-oxidation of SH groups. The major product isolated from the reactive mixture following chromatography is always the $F(ab')_2$ heterodimer (50–70%). Hybrid molecules have been constructed with equal efficiency from a range of antibodies including mouse, rat and rabbit.

We believe that thioether-linked $F(ab')_2$ derivatives are well designed to recruit cellular effectors and to deliver cytotoxic agents to unwanted cells. They are straightforward to prepare, contain only heterodimers and are completely stable to reduction. Their lack of an Fc region will prevent interaction with Fc receptor-bearing cells. This may be important, first because it avoids clearance by the reticuloendothelial system, and also because Fc regions of antibodies are able to promote antigenic modulation by binding to Fc receptors on cells such as monocytes [23] (see above), with the result that both target and effector cells become stripped of their specific antigens. In any immunotherapy which relies on the recruitment of natural effectors by antibody such clearance is best avoided [11]. More recently, Clark and Waldmann [55] have demonstrated an additional disadvantage with bispecific antibody which carry Fc regions, that is their ability to display Fc regions on effector cells which then places the effectors themselves at risk of becoming targets in K-cell-mediated ADCC. Clearly an $F(ab')_2$ bispecific antibody would not encounter this handicap and theoretically should act as nothing more than 'molecular adaptors', either giving specificity to cytotoxic agents or redirecting effector cells.

The surface Ig of neoplastic B cells has proved a highly suitable target for bispecific antibodies, promoting both the recruitment of cellular effectors and the delivery of cytotoxic agents. As with all neoplastic targets it is the use of bispecific antibodies with cellular effectors which has generated the most interest as potential therapeutic agents. In particular, bispecific antibodies look promising as one of the few derivatives capable of 'arming' cytotoxic T lymphocytes (CTLs). CTLs remain a largely untapped source of effectors in tumor therapy. However, using the appropriate bispecific antibodies it is now theoretically possible to recruit any cytotoxic T lymphocytes to destroy almost any target cell specified. Target cell specificity is controlled solely by the bispecific antibody and lysis is independent of the MHC status of the cells involved. Furthermore, the antibody does not simply glue the two cell populations together, but in linking them also provides the signal to the effector which unleashes its lytic potential. It is the molecule targeted on the effector cell which is important in providing this trigger. With CTLs, lysis can be achieved through the antigen receptor complex (usually CD3) or the 'alternative activation antigen' T11 (CD2), while lysis with LGLs occurs when binding is via the low-affinity Fc-receptor, FcRIII (CD16). Most other surface molecules found on effector cells, such as the class I MHC molecules, the CD25 antigen (IL-2 receptor) and the transferrin receptor, are unable to provide the necessary trigger [56]. While the determinant recognized on the effector is important, that recognized on the target apparently is not: surface Ig on B cells, along with many other antigens such as MHC molecules, FcR, viral antigens and various haptens on a wide range of target cells, have all proved quite suitable in directing the lytic process [46–49].

For our own studies we have recently shown that bispecific $F(ab')_2$ antibodies are powerful reagents in the recruitment of lymphokine-activated killer (LAK) cells for the destruction of B cell lymphoma. It is well documented that exposure of peripheral blood lymphocytes (PBLs) to IL-2 generates LAK cells, which are nonspecifically cytotoxic for a range of long-term cell lines and certain types of autologous tumors [57]. Although it is still unclear what cells are responsible for LAK activity, with both LGLs and CTLs probably having a role, their cytotoxic activity is such that a number of groups are using them in the treatment of late-stage malignancies [57].

We have now shown that the in vitro cytotoxic activity of LAK cells can be augmented and given target cell specificity by arming with various bispecific $F(ab')_2$ Ab. For example, LAK cells from normal donors and from tumor patients can be recruited to destroy what are normally considered LAK-resistant targets, using bispecific antibody designed to trigger either CTL (via CD3) or LGL (via CD16). Figure 4 shows such derivatives working with LAK cells from two normal donors against the lymphoblastic lymphoma line, L_2C. In this system the bispecific antibodies are binding to the targets via idiotypic determinants of the surface IgM on these cells. In the absence of antibody or with most mouse IgG isotypes (IgG3 has not been available for investigation), L_2C cells are completely resistant to LAK-mediated lysis. However, when either of the bispecific Ab, anti-CD3 × anti-idiotype or anti-CD16 × anti-idiotype, was added lysis was accomplished. We believe that the combination of LAK cells with one or more appropriate bispecific antibody could prove very effective in tumor therapy.

Bispecific antibodies, in using an antigen-binding site rather than an Fc region for the recruitment of cellular effectors, clearly have a number of theoretical advantages over conventional antibodies. In particular, they allow an increased level of selection of the effectors recruited. Derivatives

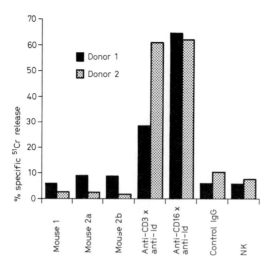

Fig. 4. Bispecific antibody for the targeting of LAKs against ^{51}Cr-labelled L_2C lymphoma cells. LAKs were generated by culturing PBLs from 2 normal donors for 5 days in IL-2. In a standard 3-h ^{51}Cr release assay LAK cells were unable to lyse the L_2C targets (NK). Furthermore, lysis was not induced by the addition of saturating levels of mouse monoclonal anti-L_2C antibody (anti-idiotype Ab) of various isotypes (γ1, γ2a or γ2b). However, effective lysis was seen when either of the two bispecific F(ab′)$_2$ Ab, anti-CD3 × anti-idiotype (anti-Id) and anti-CD16 × anti-Id, were added. These results suggest that both CTLs (OKT3$^+$) and LGLs (CD16$^+$) may be recruited from LAK cell preparations.

which rely on Fc regions will usually bind to a number of different types of Fc receptor expressed on a wide range of cells, not all of which will be useful in killing target cells. In contrast, a bispecific F(ab′)$_2$ antibody, designed to bind just one type of Fc receptor, e.g. FcRIII with the monoclonal antibody 3G8 [46], allows far more control over which effectors are activated. Furthermore, by utilizing epitopes on the receptor which lie outside its IgG-binding site, it should be possible to design bispecific antibodies which bind to the FcR in such a way that they are not hindered by nonimmune IgG, even at the concentrations found in vivo (up to 10 mg/ml). Finally, bispecific antibodies are the only derivative with the potential for recruiting large numbers of unprimed CTLs.

The use of bispecific antibodies as vectors for pharmacological agents has not been extensively investigated [51–53]. In those experiments which have been done, the surface Ig of B cells seems to offer a particularly suitable target for attack, possibly due to its readiness to be internalized, or because of the compartment into which it delivers the toxic component. Work with immunotoxins has suggested that antigens which have a tendency to modulate (e.g. the transferrin receptor and CD22 marker on B cells) are better at delivering toxic molecules such as ricin A chain into target cells than those markers which do not [58].

Raso and Griffin [51] were the first to demonstrate that $F(ab')_2$ heterodimers, in which one Fab′ arm was directed at surface Ig of the Daudi cell line and the other bound to ricin A chain, could specifically deliver the toxin to the target cells and prevent further protein synthesis. More recently we have extended this work and shown that bispecific $F(ab')_2$ can target the ribosome-inactivating protein, saporin, to unwanted cells in vivo [59]. For these experiments thioether-linked $F(ab')_2$ heterodimers were constructed with one specificity for the saporin molecule and the other for idiotypic IgM of the guinea pig lymphoblastic lymphoma, L_2C. In vitro experiments measuring protein synthesis showed that saporin was close to 90,000 times more toxic to the L_2C cells when the bispecific antibody was added to the cultures. Thus, while the concentration of free saporin needed to inhibit protein synthesis by 50% (IC_{50}) was approximately $6 \times 10^{-7} M$ (18 µg/ml), when a bispecific $F(ab')_2$ (1 µg/ml) was added the same level of inhibition could be attained with saporin at below $7 \times 10^{-12} M$ (0.21 ng/ml). This level of toxicity was very similar to that obtained with a conventional immunotoxin in which saporin was covalently linked to anti-idiotype. Direct comparison of the bispecific antibody approach with the immunotoxin (fig. 5) suggests that the bispecific antibody is at least as good and in some cases better than immunotoxin at delivering toxins to target cells in vitro. In addition, examination of the control derivatives suggests that the main advantage of a bispecific $F(ab')_2$ may lie not in its increased level of potency for target cells, but in a decreased level of nonspecific toxicity.

Bispecific $F(ab')_2$ has also performed well in tumor-bearing guinea pigs (fig. 6). A small dose of saporin (10–25 µg) which by itself showed no therapeutic effect, eradicated all detectable idiotype-positive tumor when given in combination with an excess of bispecific Ab. Although tumors did eventually emerge in most of these animals, immunofluorescence analysis shows that in almost all cases the escaping cells were idiotype negative. These cells represent rare variants of the L_2C, which persist in the wild-type population and fail to express surface Ig due to a loss of µ-chain production. Their light chain is synthesized normally [9]. This level of protection in an aggressive tumor like the L_2C, which doubles every 19 h, requires that all but

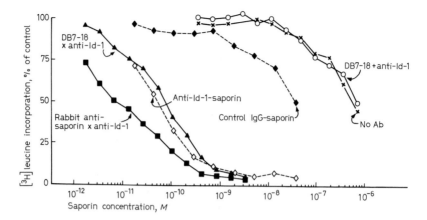

Fig. 5. Uptake of [³H]leucine by the lymphoblastic B cell leukemia L₂C, when cultured in medium containing either a mixture of bispecific antibody and saporin or a saporin-containing immunotoxin. Cells (5 × 10⁶/ml) were cultured in supplemented DMEM containing saporin at the concentration indicated plus: DMEM only (No Ab); an equal mixture of F(ab′)₂ (1 µg/ml) from DB7-18 (monoclonal antisaporin) + anti-Id-1; bispecific F(ab′)₂DB7-18 × anti-idiotype-1 (anti-Id-1) (1 µg/ml); or bispecific F(ab′)₂ rabbit antisaporin × anti-Id-1 (1 µg/ml). Parallel cultures contained the immunotoxins, control IgG-saporin and anti-Id-1-saporin (saporin at the concentration indicated), in which the saporin was disulfide bonded to the immunoglobulin using SPDP [9]. After 8 h at 37 °C cultures were pulsed with [³H]leucine for a further 12 h before harvesting the incorporated radioactivity. The most striking observation is that adding bispecific F(ab′)₂ to cell cultures can significantly enhance the toxicity of saporin. For the rabbit Fab′-containing derivative, this has resulted in almost a 100,000-fold shift in the toxicity of saporin for L₂C.

a minute proportion of the tumor inoculum be destroyed by treatment. Indeed, based on this doubling time, it is possible to calculate that perhaps less than five cells have escaped to seed the emerging tumor.

Experiments to define the optimal treatment regimen in this model have shown that, while the administration of saporin and bispecific antibody at separate sites can be therapeutically effective, mixing the antibody and saporin to form immune complexes prior to injection usually enhances their performance [59]. Similarly, when using small doses of saporin, a molar surplus of antibody (at least 3:1) is generally required in these mixtures for optimum treatment. Our current immunotherapy model, in which guinea pigs are first inoculated with 10⁵ L₂C cells on day 0, treated on day 1 and then observed for survival, has failed to distinguish whether the combination of

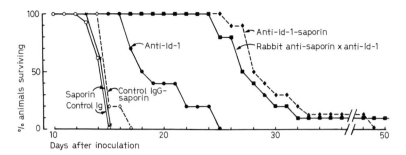

Fig. 6. Immunotherapy with a mixture of saporin and bispecific F(ab')₂ or immuno-toxin. Groups of guinea pigs (at least 9 in each) were inoculated intraperitoneally with 10^5 L_2C cells (day 0). After 24 h they were given a single treatment i.p. as indicated and survival was recorded. Animals in the various groups were given: control IgG (1 mg); anti-Id-1 IgG (1 mg); saporin only (30 µg); control IgG-saporin (140 µg: saporin content 30 µg); anti-Id-1-saporin (140 µg: saporin content 30 µg); and a mixture of bispecific F(ab')₂ (125 µg of rabbit antisaporin × anti-Id-1) and saporin (25 µg). All tumors emerging in the animals treated with anti-Id-1-saporin or the mixture of bispecific F(ab')₂ and saporin were Id-negative variants of the L_2C.

bispecific antibody and saporin can be more effective than the conventional immunotoxin. Both strategies have given similar levels of protection and been thwarted by the emergence of the idiotype-negative variants. With further work, using more demanding therapeutic regimens, it should be possible to make this distinction.

Theoretically, the delivery of toxins with bispecific antibody could have a number of advantages over the more conventional immunoconjugates. First, bispecific derivatives can be prepared without any chemical modification to the antibody binding sites or the toxic compound, thus ensuring that both components remain biologically active. Second, because bispecific Ab, unlike most immunoconjugates, can be constructed precisely without the use of lysine-reactive cross-linkers, we can expect a high level of reproducibility in their performance. Third, by using Abs which sterically hinder any ligand-binding activity a cytotoxic agent might have, e.g. the galactose-binding sites on ricin, it may be possible to reduce or block toxicity of the agent to normal tissues, while maintaining specific delivery to the unwanted cells via the second antibody specificity. Fourth, no covalent bond need be broken to release the toxic substance once the complex has bound and entered a target cell. Finally, the drop in pH experienced by complexes following their internalization into the endosomal compartment of the cell should encourage the dissociation of complexes and give the cytotoxic agent maximum opportunity to cross into the cytosol and destroy the target cell.

The major disadvantage for bispecific antibodies as vectors for cytotoxic agents in vivo would appear to be their reliance on comparatively weak, reversible interactions for maintaining union between the carrier and ligand until the target cell is reached and entered. Our preliminary investigations in vivo using bispecific antibody to target saporin show that targeting is most effective using a molar excess of the Ab. Presumably under these conditions toxin which becomes detached from antibody during delivery rapidly reunites with fresh antibody before it can be excreted. Most bispecific derivatives are also univalent for the target cell. Not only will this reduce affinity for the target antigen, it could also prevent uptake into cells by antigenic modulation which usually requires a bivalent ligand to cross-link cell surface antigens. However, many univalent ligands, including antibody Fab' fragments, do gain entry into cells [60] probably as a result of constitutive turnover or recycling of the target antigen in the plasma membrane.

It will take extensive testing in a number of model systems before we will know if the theoretical advantages of a bispecific antibody approach can offset its apparent disadvantages when targeting cytotoxic agents. As yet we have not found a significant difference between bispecific antibody and immunotoxin for targeting in vivo. The results obtained with bispecific $F(ab')_2$ in the L_2C-bearing guinea pigs have been surprisingly good, and consequently we shall continue to investigate both approaches until clear differences can be identified.

Antigen-Primed B Cells as Targets for Cytotoxic T Lymphocytes

The interaction between antigen-primed antigen-presenting cells (APC), such as macrophages and dendritic cells, and helper T cells (CD4) is generally considered an inductive phase of the immune response in which help is supplied to B cells and other T cells [61–63]. Recently, however, a number of groups have shown that, in vitro at least, once an APC has been primed with antigen it becomes susceptible to lysis by cloned antigen-specific helper T cells [64–67]. The kinetics of cytolysis appeared to parallel other features of T cell activation such as IL-2 production and proliferation. Furthermore, unlike conventional T cell cytotoxicity which is mediated by CD8+ cells and is class I restricted, this lysis is class II restricted and most if not all cloned T helper cells are active. In fact, the frequency with which cloned helper T cells display lytic activity has prompted Ju et al [67] to suggest that if a similar activity were to occur in vivo, then it would provide a mechanism for immunosuppression in which APC activity would decay as a result of lysis of APC following T cell-APC interaction.

Recent experiments have now shown that B cells can also process and present antigen on their class II molecules in much the same way as other APC such as macrophages and dendritic cells [61]. However, unlike conventional APC, which acquire antigen nonspecifically, B cells use their surface Ig to recognize and internalize soluble antigen making the process vastly more efficient [68]. The question of how important B cell processing is in driving those cells into full antibody production during an immune response remains to be answered.

The implications of these two areas of research for therapy of neoplastic B cells has now been investigated by Ochi et al. [69], who have shown that if antigen is conjugated to anti-idiotype it can be delivered to the appropriate neoplastic B cell, where it is processed and presented to antigen-specific cytotoxic T cells. In this system keyhole limpet hemocyanin (KLH) was conjugated to anti-idiotype and once again the KLH-specific cytotoxic T cells were of the CD4 helper phenotype, making the killing class II restricted. Lanzavecchia et al. [70] have modified and extended this work to show that the mouse monoclonal antibody itself can be used as the target antigen for class-II-restricted T cell. This maneuver does away with the need for any antibody-antigen conjugate. Furthermore, the antibody does not have to recognize the surface Ig of the B cell lymphoma. Antibodies binding to other, and probably all surface antigens, including class II, β_2-microglobulin, transferrin receptor and CD21, will also prime neoplastic B cells for cytolysis. This latter observation suggests that the approach need not be restricted to anti-idiotype antibodies and could employ xenogenic antibodies against a range of TAAs on any class II-positive tumor.

The major attraction of this strategy is that it exploits properties, such as antigen processing and presentation, which are presumably inherent in the B cell. Antigenic modulation should help and not hinder any attempt at therapy. Furthermore, unlike antibody and antibody derivatives which are only active for a relatively short period while they remain at the cell surface, processed antigen stays in and on B cells for extended periods so they remain sensitive to specific CTLs for at least 24 h at 37 °C. In some investigations [67] APC do not become fully sensitive to lysis until after 20 h of exposure to antigen.

However, this approach is not without its difficulties for in vivo applications, probably the major one being that of generating a specific CTL response. If it is intended that the response should be generated in vivo, then it will be difficult, although perhaps not impossible [71], to produce a strong T cell response in the absence of an antibody response. Antibodies would block access of an antigen to the tumor in much the same way that idiotypic Ig can prevent anti-idiotype reaching a B cell lymphoma, i.e. forming immune complexes which are removed via the reticuloendothelial system of the liver and spleen. Administering excess antigen in an attempt to 'mop up' the excess antibody would be unlikely to overcome the problem, since the specific focusing of T cells in this system relies on low levels of antigen [69]. At high antigen concentrations specificity is lost, presumably because when antigen is taken nonspecifically any class II expressing cell can become a target for lysis and T cell activity would be diverted to inappropriate targets.

An alternative approach which might be considered would be to immunize not with an intact antigen, but with fragments of antigen which are normally buried in the native structure. Having produced an immune response, including both T and B cell components, to such fragments, the patient would then receive the native antigen perhaps coupled to a targeting antibody such as anti-idiotype. The native antigen would not be recognized by antibodies because the immunizing fragment(s) would be buried, but after processing and presentation by the class II-positive target cells, these hidden determinants would be made available to specific CTL. One could perhaps consider using a nonpathological virus for such work, immunizing with internal proteins such as nuclear protein to produce a delayed-type hypersensitivity response, and then delivering the intact virus [72]. Finally, there is the question of whether it will be possible or necessary to generate a class II-restricted cytotoxic T cell response. Germain [63] has suggested that antigen taken up from the fluid phase or by receptor-mediated endocytosis from outside the APC, always end up associated with class II, while peptides produced from proteins residing in the cytoplasm, such as those produced by viruses, are carried to the cell surface in class I molecules. If correct, this hypothesis suggests that extraneous antigens which are delivered to target cells for processing will only be available to class II-restricted cells, and that cytotoxic class II-restricted T cells will be a necessary requirement of this approach.

Generation of Active Anti-Idiotypic Immunity

An alternative approach to the passive administration of antibody or antibody derivatives is to actively immunize with the tumor-derived idiotypic Ig, in order to generate an anti-idiotypic immune response in the patient or the experimental animal. Such an approach has the advantage over passive immunotherapy that the anti-tumor response, once generated, will be present on a continuing basis. This means that such an approach may be particularly useful in dealing with residual disease following debulking of the tumor either by passive antibody therapy or by more conventional forms of treatment. Active immunization with idiotypic Ig, as will be discussed below, was first demonstrated using murine plasmacytomas, and has more recently been extended to lymphomas which secrete little Ig.

Plasmacytomas

The murine plasmacytomas have proved invaluable as models for the study of Ig-secreting tumors [73] although it has to be said that there is no clear counterpart to this group of tumors in human proliferative disease. The vast majority of human neoplasms of secreting plasma cells, the multiple myelomas, differ from the murine plasmacytomas in failing to express Ig at the cell surface. This presumably means that immune attack or suppression of such cells by anti-idiotypic pathways cannot operate, although a postulated less mature precursor cell theoretically would be susceptible [74]. In any case it is difficult to envisage a therapeutic application to any tumor which secretes comparatively large amounts of idiotypic Ig, even if it is also expressed at the cell surface. Current chemotherapeutic schedules capable of reducing tumor load to levels where immunization could be contemplated would undoubtedly also reduce the capacity of the immune system to respond.

In spite of these disadvantages of the murine model, the tumors have provided a great deal of information on plasma cell differentiation in vivo and on responses of mature B cells to immunoregulatory signals [73]. They also provided a source of secreted idiotypic Ig which could be purified and used to immunize mice prior to tumor challenge. Results indicated that such immunization induced protective antitumor responses in a number of the plasmacytomas [75], and opened up the study of mechanisms of tumor suppression [73]. The protection obtained against tumor development after an intensive prior immunization schedule with idiotypic Ig was significant for several of the plasmacytomas and particularly strong for MOPC 315 [73]. Importantly, the protection was shown to be idiotype specific and a proportion of tumors emerging in immunized mice appeared to be variants which failed to express idiotypic Ig [75].

Lymphomas

A better therapeutic target is presented by the B cell leukemias and lymphomas, the majority of which express Ig at the cell surface and secrete comparatively little or no Ig [76]. In the past, this led to difficulty in obtaining sufficient idiotypic Ig for purification and immunization, but recent techniques whereby tumor cells from either mouse or human sources, after hybridization to a suitable myeloma-derived fusion partner can be made to secrete idiotypic Ig, have largely surmounted this problem [77]. Preimmunization with idiotypic IgM has been shown to be protective against subsequent tumor challenge for the L_2C leukemia of guinea pigs [78] and also against two mouse B cell lymphomas [79, 80]. In all cases, the protection was idiotype specific, suggesting that anti-idiotypic responses are effective against a range of B cell tumors.

Our studies have focused on the mouse B cell lymphoma, BCL_1, first described by Slavin and Strober [81] and used previously as a model for antibody-toxin therapy [82]. The lymphoma has a preferential localization in the spleen and has been compared to human prolymphocytic leukemia [83]. Tumor cells express $IgM\lambda$, together with a small amount of $IgD\lambda$, quite strongly at the cell surface, and secrete low levels of idiotypic IgM [84]. For an animal lymphoma, the division rate is relatively low, with a doubling time of approximately 3 days [83]. Mice passaged with a large inoculum of cells (5×10^5) die in 38 ± 10 days: lower cell doses can increase survival time although a single cell is capable of inducing lethal tumor [83]. Idiotypic IgM was obtained by hybridization of the tumor cells to a myeloma line, and the pentameric IgM purified and used to immunize BALB/c mice with complete Freund's adjuvant [79]. The protocol adopted was a primary injection of 50 µg of IgM in two subcutaneous sites, followed by boosts after 3 and 4 weeks. This amount of IgM was found to be effective in the plasmacytoma model [73] and has been used in other lymphoma models [78, 80]. Tumor cells (5×10^5) were injected i.p. 1 week after the final boost and the mice were observed. Protection induced was clear and specific, with 70/90 animals surviving >100 days, as compared to controls (38 ± 10 days). This degree of protection is greater than that induced by a similar schedule in the L_2C leukemia [78] or in the chemically induced mouse B cell lymphoma 38C13 [80]: in the latter it was necessary to link the idiotypic IgM to the immunogenic carrier KLH to generate an effective antitumor response and challenge doses were generally low (200 cells). The reason for the great effectiveness of immunization in the BCL_1 tumor is not known although its relatively low division rate, more in keeping with human disease [83], might be a factor.

Attempts to treat tumor-bearing mice by active immunization are limited by the short time available to generate an immune response, during which tumor growth proceeds unimpeded. In the BCL_1 lymphoma it has been

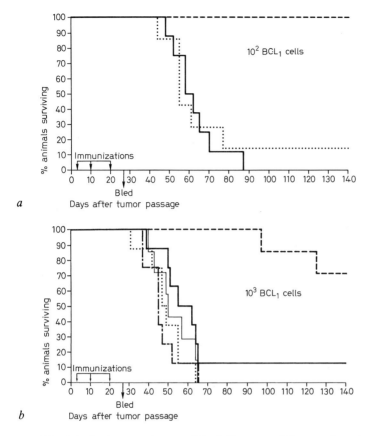

Fig. 7. Active immunotherapy of the BCL$_1$ tumor. Mice were inoculated with 10^2 or 10^3 BCL$_1$ cells and immunized with: BCL$_1$ IgM (——); BCL$_1$ IgM-KLH (---); MOPC 104E IgM, (——); MOPC 104E IgM-KLH (—·—), or left unimmunized (····). The animals were tail bled on day 27 and their survival noted.

possible to treat mice passaged with 10^2 or 10^3 tumor cells by instituting immunization 3 days post passage [85]. In this necessarily artificial model, immunization with idiotypic IgM linked to KLH was very effective (fig. 7), but if the tumor dose was raised to 10^4 cells, only a slight effect was seen. If the antigen was not linked to KLH, the immune response generated was ineffective, and this could be due to the slower rate of induction of the response as evidenced by serum anti-idiotypic antibody (fig. 8). It is the rate of induction rather than the final antibody titer which appears to be the major factor in successful therapy [85]: this is dealt with more fully below.

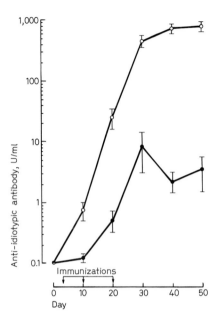

Fig. 8. Induction of anti-idiotypic immune response. Mice were immunized with either BCL_1 IgM-KLH (○) or BCL_1 IgM (●), tail bled every 10 days and the serum samples assayed for anti-idiotypic antibody. The results are expressed as the mean ± SEM of 8 animals.

Mechanisms of Anti-Idiotypic Immunity

One difficulty in assessing the role of the various effector mechanisms in the anti-idiotypic immunity clearly evident in immunized animals is the fact that experiments in vitro are necessarily artificial and may be misleading. For this reason, the section is subdivided into results obtained in vivo, and those demonstrable in vitro but not necessarily relevant in the whole animal.

Involvement of Humoral and Cellular Responses in vivo

Passive Transfer Studies

In order to demonstrate clear involvement of the humoral or cellular immune response in protection against tumor development, passive transfer studies are required. Thus, in unimmunized recipient animals it should be possible to inject a tumor challenge together with either antibody or cells obtained from animals previously immunized with idiotypic Ig, and then to observe suppression of tumor development. This is not without technical difficulty, particularly for cell transfer since there is the problem of survival and appropriate localization of the injected immune cells, but a positive result is a strong indication for the involvement of that mechanism. Such an approach of adoptive immunotherapy has been used in a series of studies on a mouse virus-induced leukemia, FBL-3 [86]. In this case cytotoxic T cells were generated by immunization with irradiated tumor cells and these cells prevented tumor growth if transferred with tumor cells [86]. This at least demonstrates the feasibility of the system, but such clear results have not been obtained for the anti-idiotypic immune response. This may be partly due to the fact that anti-idiotypic cytotoxic T cells generally do not seem to be generated by immunization with purified idiotypic Ig [87]. In contrast, when irradiated plasmacytoma cells were used as immunogen, cytotoxic T cells were generated but they did not recognize idiotypic determinants [87].

In the murine plasmacytoma model, MOPC 315, a detailed investigation of the participation of the humoral and cellular responses in idiotype-specific protection against tumor was undertaken [88]. Serum from immunized mice was injected over a long period starting 3 weeks before tumor challenge, and some degree of tumor suppression was observed although it was variable. For analysis of the cellular response, adoptive transfer into irradiated hosts was used and the only protocol which was effective was to inject immune spleen cells together with a boost of idiotypic Ig, which itself could have generated antibody [88]. Thus, it was not possible to assign a major role to either antibody or cells in protection and the evidence suggested that both were required [89]. A similar failure to transfer immunity using spleen cells from mice immunized with idiotypic IgG from the MOPC 11 tumor has been reported: in this study immune serum was not tested by transfer since no cytotoxic antibody was detected in vitro [90].

The picture for the low or nonsecreting lymphomas is rather different in that for the limited number of systems investigated anti-idiotypic antibody appears to be of greater importance in protection against tumor than T cells. Perhaps a cell which expresses idiotypic Ig quite strongly but secretes little is more susceptible to antibody attack than the highly secreting plasmacytoma cell which would presumably rapidly neutralize antibody in its vicinity. The B cell lymphomas which have been investigated are the L_2C leukemia of strain 2 guinea pigs, where cytotoxic anti-idiotypic antibody was demonstrated [78] and the murine B cell lymphomas BCL_1 and 38C13 [79, 80]. For BCL_1, passive transfer studies indicated a role for anti-idiotypic antibody in protection with no evidence for involvement of T cells [79]. The system used was a modified Winn assay where tumor cells were mixed with splenocytes from immunized mice and injected in an intramuscular site, but no protection was seen unless antibody was injected i.p.

The Role of Anti-Idiotypic Antibody

As indicated above, the role of syngeneic anti-idiotypic antibody in protection against tumor has been revealed for the mouse lymphoma BCL_1 by passive transfer experiments [79]. However, it is rather difficult to dissect out the therapeutic importance of the various subclasses of syngeneic antibodies. Presumably, syngeneic antiserum contains multiple anti-idiotypic antibodies of various specificities and subclasses and these could act together synergistically or competitively within the various effector systems. Some insight has been provided by the 38C13 lymphoma where individual syngeneic monoclonal anti-idiotypic antibodies of different subclasses were tested for immunotherapeutic efficacy [91]. It was found that the IgG2a subclass was particularly effective and since this subclass mediates antibody-dependent cellular cytotoxicity (ADCC), participation of this mechanism in protection has been suggested [91]. Administered xenogeneic anti-idiotypic antibodies have been shown to be effective to varying degrees against plasmacytomas [92] and lymphomas [93] but this does not necessarily support a role for antibody in the syngeneic system. In the BCL_1 model, mice immunized with idiotypic IgM generated a range of anti-idiotypic antibody levels in the serum as measured by both immunofluorescence [79] and ELISA techniques [85], and pooled antisera showed good cytotoxicity against tumor cells in the presence of fresh rat serum as a complement source [79]. However, there was no simple correlation between the levels of serum anti-idiotype immediately before tumor passage and survival time. This lack of correlation was even more marked when the idiotypic IgM was conjugated to KLH to render it a more effective antigen. In this case the serum anti-idiotypic antibody levels were clearly higher than for IgM alone, but survival times on tumor passage were indistinguishable (fig. 9) [85]. The reason for this finding appears to be the emergence of immunoresistant variants which no longer express surface idiotypic IgM: thus, a minimal level of antibody is probably effective in removing the idiotype-expressing tumor cells, after which the antibody response is beating uselessly against variant tumors [10].

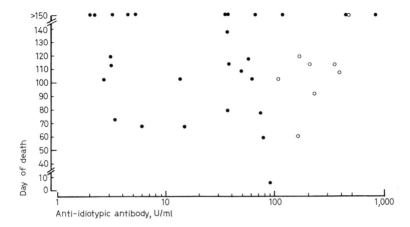

Fig. 9. Lack of correlation between anti-idiotypic antibody levels and survival. Mice were immunized with either BCL$_1$ IgM-KLH (○) or BCL$_1$ IgM (●) challenged with 5×10^5 BCL$_1$ cells and their survival noted. Before tumor challenge the animals were bled and the levels of serum anti-idiotypic antibody measured.

The time when KLH conjugation of antigen was useful was during attempts to treat mice already bearing lymphoma by active immunization. In this case speed of induction of the antibody response is critical as there is a danger of tumor growth outstripping the development of an immune response, and the conjugated antigen was more effective (see above).

The Role of Anti-Idiotypic T Cells.

Although early experiments in the MOPC 315 system indicated a role for the thymus in anti-idiotypic immunity against the plasmacytoma [73], it has proved difficult to work out the details of T cell involvement by manipulations in vivo, as has been discussed above. However, there is a wealth of data gathered in vitro which point out some possible mechanisms by which T cells could suppress tumor. In the case of the B cell lymphomas, even if T cells are not able to act directly against tumor, they must at least be involved in helping B cells to produce anti-idiotypic antibody, and it has been possible in two models to demonstrate T cells which recognize tumor-derived idiotypic IgM [79, 80]. Experiments which examine the properties of anti-idiotypic T cells in vitro are described in the following section.

Anti-Idiotypic T Cells Identified in vitro

As already indicated, there is evidence for involvement of T cells in growth suppression of the Ig-secreting tumors, with directly cytotoxic T cells rarely being reported. In the model studied in most detail, the MOPC 315 tumor, a consistent finding in vitro is that proliferation and differentiation of the tumor cells can be regulated by idiotype-specific suppressor T cells or a soluble factor derived from them [73]. These cells are Lyt-1⁻2⁺ and appear to recognize idiotypic determinants present on the variable region of the α-heavy chain of the M315 protein. Their mode of action is to suppress biosynthesis and subsequent secretion of idiotypic IgA via inhibition of synthesis of mRNA for the λ-light chain [94]. Although the heavy chain is transcribed normally, the failure of λ-chain synthesis prevents production of the secreted IgA: curiously, membrane IgA expression is not affected [94]. It is not clear what the relationship of these anti-idiotypic T_s cells which appear to affect Ig synthesis by tumor cells is to those of similar phenotype which suppress delayed-type hypersensitivity (DTH) against the myeloma protein M315 [95]. The latter T_s cells have been generated by intravenous injection of syngeneic mice with either M315-coupled splenocytes or with the F_v (V_H and V_L) fragment of M315. This cell population is also able to directly suppress IgA secretion by the myeloma cells but so far has not been found to be able to proliferate in response to idiotypic Ig in vitro, nor have the cells been grown as lines or clones. Also, the demonstration of their involvement in the regulation of myeloma growth and function in vivo has not so far been reported. In a separate study, mice injected with the light chain of M315 prior to sensitization with the whole Ig molecule again showed marked suppression of DTH to the M315 idiotype [96]. The specificity of this T cell suppressor pathway was very fine involving amino acids in the third hyper-variable loop of the L315 V domain, in the same region as that recognized by helper T cell (T_h clones (see below) [96]).

There have been several reports of helper T lymphocytes elicited by immunization with myeloma proteins [97]. In detailed studies on the specificity of recognition of the M315 protein, idiotopes present on the denatured variable domains of the α-chain or the $λ_2$-chain present in the IgA molecule were shown to be implicated [98, 99]. The latter cells might be important in suppression of tumor since mice immunized with free λ-chain or the variable region domain show idiotype-specific resistance to challenge with MOPC 315 cells [100]. Peptide analysis has indicated that a sequence from the $Vλ_2$ representing amino acid region 88-117 primed T_h cells for response to Fab derived from M315 [101] and further investigation demonstrated that T_h cells could discriminate between two λ_2-chains that differ by two amino acids at the $V\lambda_2$-$J\lambda_2$ junction [97]. Idiotope-specific T_h cell lines and clones which recognized $V\lambda_2315$, again in the third hypervariable region, have been established [101]. These cells were able to respond to Fab315 but a much greater concentration was required than for $V\lambda_2315$, suggesting that the cells, in contrast to anti-idiotypic antibody, responded preferentially to processed antigen [101]. An idiotype-specific T_h cell clone has recently been established for the mouse myeloma ABPC 48. Interestingly, the T cells responded more readily in ^{3}H-TdR incorporation assays to idiotype-positive tumor cells than to soluble antigen [102].

For the lymphomas, T cells which responded specifically to idiotypic IgM derived from tumor have been demonstrated in the spleens of mice immunized with purified IgM from both the BCL_1 and the 38C13 tumors [79, 80]. In a rather different model system, a B cell hybridoma which expresses and secretes an antiphthalate antibody and carries a private idiotype was propagated as a tumor in BALB/c mice [103]. Idiotype-specific effector T cells of Lyt-1$^+$ and Lyt-2$^-$ phenotype could be isolated from primed mice, and such cells were able to suppress both the membrane and secreted form of idiotypic Ig either in vivo or in vitro. Suppression in this case required cell contact and the mechanism involved appeared to be via induction or selection of preexisting negative mutants from the hybridoma population [104].

Dormant Tumor

The presence of dormant tumor in animals and human patients [105] has intrigued immunologists for many years, but there is still little understanding of how such dormancy is maintained. Some evidence for dormancy in the BCL_1 lymphoma was obtained during experiments to test the efficacy of treatment with anti-δ-immunotoxin [106]. Long-term survivors were examined for the presence of tumor by transferring cells from various tissues into normal recipients. Tumors did arise in these mice suggesting that the immunotoxin had not killed all target cells and that prolonged remission may be mediated by the host [106]. A similar dormant state could be induced by active immunization with idiotypic IgM [79]. In this case mice surviving for >6 months after tumor challenge with no overt sign of tumor were investigated for the presence of tumor cells in the spleen both by immunohistology and by transfer into unimmunized recipients. In three immune mice examined the spleens were normal in size and appearance but tumor cells could be detected by staining tissue sections with anti-idiotypic antibody. The numbers of idiotype-positive cells estimated from the sections were 50, 35 and 2% of total cells with residual cells being largely T cells. The tumor cells therefore appeared to be in an appropriate site. On passage of the spleen cells into 3 recipients, all developed idiotype-positive tumor in 41, 41 and 29 days. Thus, the spleens of long-term survivors can contain substantial numbers of tumor cells, apparently held in check by a mechanism which is disrupted on passage to normal recipients.

Escape of Tumor from Anti-Idiotypic Control

Modes of Escape

The ability of target tumor cells to escape from attack by either passive or active immunotherapy is an impressive adaptive phenomenon. In the case of anti-idiotypic suppression of lymphoma the cells can outmaneuver antibody and effector mechanisms by two broad strategies. The first is a temporary one whereby idiotype and its attached antibody are removed from the cell surface before the appropriate effector can act. Such a so-called temporary modulation can continue during cell division in vivo but will reverse on removal of antibody [78]. The use of modified nonmodulating antibodies can assist in circumventing this problem and has been discussed earlier. The second strategy is a more permanent one which involves immunoselection from what presumably must be a heterogeneous tumor population. For treatment with monoclonal anti-idiotypic antibody, this can mean outgrowth of cells with different idiotopes [5] whereas for treatment by active immunization the selective process can only give rise to variants which display none of the immunogenic idiotype of the immunizing Ig. The first category of idiotope variants has been described for human [5], guinea pig [9] and mouse [107] lymphomas and will be discussed in detail in another chapter in this volume. The second category of variants which are usually surface Ig negative have arisen in mouse plasmacytoma and in our studies on active immunization of the BCL_1 lymphoma and will be discussed below.

There is little information available on the mechanisms by which such variants are selected in vivo, especially in the case of active immunization where both antibody and T cells could be involved. In the study of the B cell hybrid (2C3E1) mentioned previously, generation of variants, which was noted to occur spontaneously in vivo, has been carried out in vitro using appropriately primed spleen cells and is apparently mediated by T cells of the T_h phenotype [104]. The resulting variants were initially heterogeneous but stabilized after culture and were characterized by loss of both surface and secreted idiotypic Ig. Thus, immunoselection can apparently be mediated by either antibody or T cells.

Surface Immunoglobulin-Negative Variants

The emergence of surface Ig-negative variants in mice preimmunized with idiotypic Ig and then exposed to tumor was first observed for the MOPC 315 plasmacytoma [75]. Such variants appeared to fail to synthesize the α-heavy chain of the IgA so that only λ-light chain was synthesized and secreted. Since the MOPC 315 was known to be a heterogeneous tumor with preexisting variants, the emergence of the surface Ig-negative subset was not surprising [73]. For the in vivo BCL_1 tumor the incidence of surface Ig-negative variants in the tumor population is not known, although superficial examination by immunofluorescence would suggest that such cells represent a very small percentage. Since the two negative variants which have been isolated (see below) both show a division rate lower than that of the original BCL_1 tumor cells, such variants must continue to arise spontaneously as otherwise they would be eliminated from the population. During the experiments where mice were immunized with idiotypic IgM and escaping tumors were obtained, it became clear that some of these were apparently negative for surface Ig as judged by the fluorescence-activated cell sorter (FACS) (<10% of the fluorescence showed by parental tumor) [10]. However, if these were passaged into mice at high cell numbers (5×10^5 per mouse) almost invariably a surface IgM idiotype-positive tumor resulted. Only when 10 cells were passaged was it possible to isolate stable negative variants and the two obtained have been characterized.

The two variants (known as SNAG-1 and CIN) are similar in expressing MHC class I and II antigens at levels indistinguishable from the parental BCL_1 tumor, and also in expressing Fc receptors [10]. The SNAG-1 tumor, however, although expressing idiotypic IgM at <10% of the BCL_1 cells, does contain it within the cytoplasm [10], whereas CIN has no detectable IgM. However, although the SNAG-1 variant cells are clearly capable of synthesizing idiotypic IgM which is composed of μ- and λ-chains of the same apparent molecular weight as those from parental IgM, it fails to insert it into the membrane or secrete the low levels characteristic of the BCL_1 tumor [10]. Thus, if a structural change in the protein is present, it must be quite subtle and studies are being undertaken to analyze this further. Another interesting feature of this variant is that it no longer responds to lipopolysaccharide (LPS) by either proliferation or secretion of IgM in the way in which parental tumor does, suggesting either a coincidental loss of a second receptor or linkage of LPS responsiveness to the surface expression of IgM. The third change noted in the SNAG-1 tumor is in the tumor localization in vivo. BCL_1 is a known spleen-seeking tumor and it is thought that cell division occurs in the spleen [83], with involvement of other organs only late in disease. The SNAG-1 variant, however, shows no particular preference for the spleen and the bulk of tumor at death is generally in the liver [10]. Finally, the rate of cell division is lower and consequent survival time longer for this variant. Thus, this variant tumor which differs from BCL_1 failing to express or secrete idiotypic IgM has a co-ordinate loss of LPS responsiveness, a change in organ distribution and a reduced rate of division. Recent experiments have revealed a failure of the variant to respond to IL-5, which again suggests a major change in growth control [George, unpubl. observ.]. The second variant (CIN) is rather less well characterized but appears to have more major mutational changes in the DNA coding the μ gene [manuscript in preparation]. Interestingly, this variant has also lost the ability to respond to LPS and has an organ distribution similar to the SNAG-1 variant, suggesting that the changes in the latter are not coincidental but may be linked to Ig expression.

Implications for Treatment of Human Disease

Since the idea of using idiotypic Ig as a target for immunotherapeutic attack on B cell tumors, there has been the usual fluctuation in optimism which attends any new approach. After a first apparent success of monoclonal anti-idiotypic antibody treatment for human lymphoma [3] numerous difficulties have been identified and many have been overcome [4]. The use of engineered antibodies, either univalent bispecific [11] or immunotoxins [20] now holds out real hope of reducing tumor load to background levels. However, it remains unlikely that tumor will be completely ablated by passive therapy and the addition of active immunotherapy might lead to the host being able to control residual tumor indefinitely. It is of course possible to institute active immunotherapy independent of passive antibody, provided that any previous therapy or the disease itself has not reduced the ability of the host to mount an effective immune response. The first step will be to select appropriate patients: the most suitable would probably be those with B cell low-grade follicular lymphoma. This is a relatively indolent disease with a median survival of about 7 years, a figure unaltered by chemotherapy, thus affording adequate time for the immunization to induce an effective immune response. The neoplastic cells secrete little Ig [76], therefore there would be no significant extracellular barrier to the immune effectors, yet they express surface Ig, which can act as a target. The disease also frequently waxes and wanes spontaneously, suggesting that some form of inadequate tumor regulation may be occurring [108].

Selection of a suitable adjuvant is the next step and those immediately available for human use are aluminum salts, onto which antigen is absorbed, although a wide range of other adjuvants is being developed.

Results in the mouse lymphomas indicate that immunization can suppress tumor for a long period [10] and this could be adequate for most human tumors where division rate is considerably less than for the long-passaged animal tumors. Nevertheless, the possibility of outgrowth of escaping tumors remains. If, however, as suggested by results in the BCL_1 tumor, surface Ig turns out to be involved in determining the rate of growth in vivo, the immunoselected tumors may pose less of a threat than anticipated.

Summary

Idiotypic determinants of the Ig expressed by the majority of B cell tumors present an attractive target for immunotherapeutic manipulations. The idiotypic Ig is molecularly defined and the behavior of the target cells placed under anti-idiotypic attack might have broader implications for cancer immunotherapy. Simple administration of monoclonal antibody reactive with these determinants clearly has only a limited effect on tumor load, due largely to the multiplicity of strategies by which the tumor cell can avoid such attack. These include modulation, change in idiotypic determinants due to somatic mutation, and complete loss of expression at the cell surface. If the first antibody treatment can be made more effective, for example by tailoring molecules to recruit available effector mechanisms more efficiently, or by the use of antibodies capable of delivering a lethal hit via a toxin, the tumor cell will presumably have less opportunity to escape.

A second strategy is to immunize the tumor-bearing host with idiotypic Ig obtained from tumor cells. Once in place, such an immune response should suppress tumor growth on a continuing basis. In animal lymphoma, this approach appears to prolong survival although some of the escape mechanisms encountered for passive antibody therapy are apparently operative for active therapy. Study of these mechanisms should allow insight into how cells control expression of idiotypic determinants at the cell surface and open the possibility of further therapeutic intervention. A combined approach to the treatment of human lymphoma might be envisaged whereby tumor load is reduced by passive antibody, thus leaving the immune system relatively unscathed, and even perhaps releasing natural antitumor responses which could be further stimulated by immunization.

Acknowledgments

We are indebted to our colleague George Stevenson for helpful discussions. Our work is supported by Tenovus and the Leukaemia Research Fund, U.K. Andrew George is a Beit Memorial Fellow. We thank Pauline Hutchins and Mary Moore for typing the manuscript.

References

1 Jerne, N.K.: Towards a network theory of the immune system. Ann. Immunol., Paris *125C:* 373–389 (1974).
2 Hamblin, T.J.; Abdul-Ahad, A.K.; Gordon, J.; Stevenson, F.K.; Stevenson, G.T.: Preliminary experience in treating lymphocytic leukaemia with antibody to immunoglobulin idiotypes on the cell surfaces. Br. J. Cancer *42:* 495–502 (1980).
3 Miller, R.A.; Maloney, D.G.; Warnke, R.; Levy, R.: Treatment of B-cell lymphoma with monoclonal anti-idiotype antibody. New Engl. J. Med. *306:* 517–522 (1982).
4 Gordon, J.; Abdul-Ahad, A.K.; Hamblin, T.J.; Stevenson, F.K.; Stevenson, G.T.: Mechanisms of tumour cell escape encountered in treating lymphocytic leukaemia with anti-idiotypic antibody. Br. J. Cancer *49:* 547–557 (1984).
5 Meeker, T.; Lowder, J.; Cleary, M.L.; Stewart, S.; Warnke, R.; Sklar, J.; Levy, R.: Emergence of idiotype variants during treatment of B-cell lymphoma with anti-idiotype antibodies. New Engl. J. Med. *312:* 1658–1665 (1985).
6 Glennie, M.J.; Stevenson, G.T.: Univalent antibodies kill tumour cells in vitro and in vivo. Nature, Lond. *295:* 712–714 (1982).
7 Glennie, M.J.; McBride, H.M.; Worth, A.T.; Stevenson, G.T.: Preparation and performance of bispecific F(ab')$_2$ antibody containing thioether-linked Fab' fragments. J. Immun. *139:* 2367–2375 (1987).
8 Meeker, T.C.; Lowder, J.; Maloney, D.G.; Miller, R.A.; Thielemans, K.; Warnke, R.; Levy, R.: A clinical trial of anti-idiotypic therapy for B cell malignancy. Blood *65:* 1349–1363 (1985).
9 Glennie, M.J.; McBride, H.M.; Stirpe, F.; Thorpe, P.E.; Worth, A.T.; Stevenson, G.T.: Emergence of immunoglobulin variants following treatment of a B-cell leukemia with an immunotoxin composed of anti-idiotype and saporin. J. exp. Med. *166:* 43–62 (1987).
10 George, A.J.T.; Spellerberg, M.B.; Stevenson, F.K.: Idiotype vaccination leads to the emergence of a stable surface Ig-negative variant of the mouse lymphoma BCL$_1$, with different growth characteristics. J. Immun. *140:* 1695–1701 (1988).
11 Stevenson, G.T.; Glennie, M.J.: Surface immunoglobulin of B-lymphocytes as a therapeutic target. Cancer Surv. *4:* 213–244 (1985).
12 Gordon, J.; Stevenson, G.T.: Antigenic modulation of lymphocytic surface immunoglobulin yielding resistance to complement-mediated lysis. II. Relationship to redistribution of the antigen. Immunology *42:* 13–17 (1981).
13 Dyer, M.J.S.; Hale, G.; Hayhoe, F.G.J.; Waldemann, H.: Effects of CAMPATH-1 antibodies in vivo in patients with lymphoid malignancies: Influence of antibody isotype. Blood *July 1988.*
14 Lanier, L.L.; Babcock, G.F.; Raybourne, R.B.; Arnold, L.W.; Warner, N.L.;

Haughton, G.: Mechanism of B cell lymphoma immunotherapy with passive xeno-geneic anti-idiotype serum. J. Immun. *125:* 1730–1736 (1980).

15 Ortaldo, J.R.; Woodhorse, C.; Morgan, A.C.; Herberman, R.B.; Cheresh, D.A.; Reisfeld, R.: Analysis of effector cells in human antibody-dependent cellular cytotox-icity with murine monoclonal antibodies. J. Immun. *138:* 3566–3572 (1987).

16 Seto, M.; Takahashi, T.; Nakamura, S.; Saito, M.; Hara, T.; Nishizuka, Y.: Effector mechanism in antitumor activity of monoclonal antibodies produced against an ascitic mouse mammary tumor. Cancer Res. *46:* 2056–2061 (1986).

17 Lubeck, M.D.; Kimoto, Y.; Steplewski, Z.; Koprowski, H.: Killing of human tumor cell lines by human monocytes and murine monoclonal antibodies. Cell. Immunol. *111:* 107–117 (1988).

18 Dearman, R.J.; Stevenson, F.K.; Wrightham, M.; Hamblin, T.J.; Glennie, M,J.; Stevenson, G.T.: Lymphokine-activated killer cells from normal and lymphoma subjects are cytotoxic for cells. Blood *72:* 1985–1991 (1988).

19 Ehrlich, P.: A general review of the work in immunity; in Collected Papers of Paul Ehrlich, vol. 2. Immunology and Cancer Research, 442 (Pergamon Press, London).

20 Thorpe, P.E.: Antibody carriers of cytotoxic agents in cancer therapy; in Pinchera, Doria, Dammacco, Bargellesi, Monoclonal antibodies 84: biological and clinical applications, 475 (Editrice Kurtis SRL, Milan 1985).

21 Stevenson, G.T.; Glennie, M,J.; Paul, F.E.; Stevenson, F.K.; Watts, H.F.; Wyeth, P.: Preparation and properties of FabIgG, a chimeric univalent antibody designed to attack tumour cells. Biosci. Rep. *5:* 991–998 (1985).

22 Stevenson, G.T.; Glennie, M.J.; Hamblin, T.J.; Lane, A.C.; Stevenson, F.K.: Prob-lems and prospects in the use of lymphoma idiotypes as therapeutic targets. Int. J. Cancer, suppl. 3 (1988).

23 Schroff, R.W.; Klein, R.A.; Farrell, M.M.; Stevenson, H.C.: Enhancing effects of monocytes on modulation of a lymphocyte membrane antigen. J. Immun. *133:* 2270–2277 (1984).

24 Gordon, J.; Robinson, D.S.F.; Stevenson, G.T.: Antigenic modulation of lympho-cytic surface immunoglobulin yielding resistance to complement-mediated lysis. Immunology *42:* 7–12 (1981).

25 Hamblin, T.J.; Cattan, A.R.; Glennie, M.J.; MacKenzie, M.R.; Stevenson, F.K.; Watts, H.F.; Stevenson, G.T.: Initial experience in treating human lymphoma with a chimeric univalent derivative of monoclonal anti-idiotype antibody. Blood *69:* 790–797 (1987).

26 Khazaeli, M.B.; Saleh, M.N.; Wheeler, R.H.; Huster, W.J.; Holden, H.; Carrano, R.; Lobuglio, A.F.: Phase I trial of multiple large doses of murine monoclonal antibody CO17-1A. II. Parmacokinetics and immune response. J. natn. Cancer Inst. *80:* 937–942 (1988).

27 Stevenson, G.T.; Pindar, A.; Slade, C.J.: Chimeric antibody with dual Fc regions (bisFabFc) prepared by manipulations at the IgG hinge. Anti-Cancer Drug Design *3:* 219–230 (1988).

28 Boulianne, G.L.; Hozumi, N.; Shulman, M.J.: Production of functional chimaeric mouse/human antibody. Nature, Lond. *312:* 643–646 (1984).

29 Morrison, S.L.; Johnson, M.J.; Herzenberg, L.A.; Oi, V.T.: Chimeric human anti-body molecules: mouse antigen-binding domains with human constant region do-mains. Proc. natn. Acad. Sci. USA *81:* 6851–6855 (1984).

30 Riechmann, L.; Clark, M.; Waldmann, H.; Winter, G.: Reshaping human antibodies for therapy. Nature, Lond. *332:* 323–327 (1988).

31 Huston, J.S.; Levinson, D.; Mudgett-Hunter, M.; Tai, M.S.; Novotny, J.; Margolies, M.N.; Ridge, R.J.; Bruccoleri, R.E.; Haber, E.; Crea, R.; Oppermann, H.: Protein engineering of antibody binding sites: Recovery of specific activity in an anti-digoxin single-chain Fv analogue produced in Escherichia coli. Proc. natn. Acad. Sci. USA *85:* 5879–5883 (1988).

32 Bruggemann, M.; Williams, G.T.; Bindon, C.I.; Clark, M.R.; Walker, M.R.; Jefferis, R.; Waldmann, H.; Neuberger, M.S.: Comparison of the effector functions of human immunoglobulins using a matched set of chimeric antibodies. J. exp. Med. *166:* 1351–1361 (1987).

33 Steplewski, Z.; Sun, L.K.; Shearman, C.W.; Ghrayeb, J.; Daddona, P.; Koprowski, H.: Biological activity of human-mouse IgG1, IgG2, IgG3, and IgG4 chimeric monoclonal antibodies with antitumor specificity. Proc. natn. Acad. Sci. USA *85:* 4852–4856 (1988).

34 Bindon, C.I.; Hale, G.; Bruggemann, M.; Waldmann, H.: Human monoclonal IgG isotypes differ in complement activating function at the level of C4 as well as C1q. J. exp. Med. *168:* 127–142 (1988).

35 Burton, D.R.: Structure and function of antibodies; in Calabi, Neuberger, Molecular genetics of immunoglobulin, pp. 1–47 (Elsevier, Oxford 1987).

36 Woof, J.M.; Partridge, L.J.; Jefferis, R.; Burton, D.R.: Localisation of the monocyte-binding region on human immunoglobulin G. Molec. Immunol. *23:* 319–330 (1986).

37 Duncan, A.R.; Woof, J.M.; Partridge, L.J.; Burton, D.; Winter, G.: Localization of the binding site for the human high-affinity Fc receptor on IgG. Nature, Lond. *332:* 563–564 (1988).

38 Duncan, A.R.; Winter, G.: The binding site for C1q on IgG. Nature, Lond. *332:* 738–740 (1988).

39 LoBuglio, A.F.: Personal commun.

40 Morell, A.; Terry, W.; Waldmann, T.: Metabolic properties of IgG subclasses in man. J. clin. Invest. *49:* 673–680 (1970).

41 Sears, H.F.; Herlyn, D.; Steplewski, Z.; Koprowski, H.: Phase II clinical trial of a murine monoclonal antibody cytotoxic for gastrointestinal adenocarcinoma. Cancer Res. *45:* 5910–5913 (1985).

42 Paulus, H.: Preparation and biomedical application of bispecific antibodies. Behrint. Inst. Mitt. *78:* 118 (1985).

43 Nisonoff, A.; Mandy, W.J.: Quantitative estimation of the hybridization of the rabbit antibodies. Nature, Lond. *194:* 355–359 (1962).

44 Milstein, C.; Cuello, A.C.: Hybrid hybridomas and their use in immunohistochemistry. Nature, Lond. *305:* 537–540 (1983).

45 Suresh, M.R.; Cuello, A.C.; Milstein, C.: Advantages of bispecific hybridomas in one-step immunocytochemistry and immunoassays. Proc. natn. Acad. Sci. USA *83:* 7989–7993 (1986).

46 Karpovsky, B.; Titus, J.A.; Stephany, D.A.; Segal, D.M.: Production of target-specific effector cells using hetero-cross-linked aggregates containing anti-target cell and anti-Fc receptor antibodies. J. exp. Med. *160:* 1686–1701 (1984).

47 Staerz, U.D.; Bevan, M.J.: Use of anti-receptor antibodies to focus T-cell activity. Immunol. Today *7:* 241–245 (1986).

48 Perez, P.; Hoffman, R.W.; Titus, J.A.; Segal, D.M.: Specific targeting of human peripheral blood T cells by heteroaggregates containing anti-T3 cross linked to anti-target cell antibodies. J. exp. Med. *163:* 166–178 (1986).

49 Lanzavecchia, A.; Scheidegger, D.: The use of hybrid hybridomas to target human cytotoxic T lymphocytes. Eur. J. Immunol. 17:105–111 (1987).

50 Titus, J.A.; Garrido, M.A.; Hecht, T.T.; Winkler, D.F.; Wunderlich, J.R.; Segal, D.M.: Human T cells targeted with anti-T3 cross-linked to antitumor antibody prevent tumor growth in nude mice. J. Immun. 138: 4018–4022 (1987).

51 Raso, V.; Griffin, T.: Hybrid antibodies with dual specificity for the delivery of ricin to immunoglobulin-bearing target cells. Cancer Res. 41: 2073–2078 (1981).

52 Webb, K.S.; Ware, J.L.; Parks, S.F.; Walther, P.J.; Paulson, D.F.: Evidence for a novel hybrid immunotoxin recognizing ricin A-chain by one antigen-combining site and a prostate-restricted antigen by the remaining antigen-combining site. Potential for immunotherapy. Cancer Treat. Rep. 69: 663–672 (1985).

53 Corvalan, J.R.F.; Smith, W.; Gore, V.A.; Brandon, D.R.: Specific in vitro and in vivo drug localisation of tumour cells using a hybrid-hybrid monoclonal antibody recognising both carcinoembryonic antigen (CEA) and vinca alkaloids. Cancer Immunol. Immunother. 24: 133–137 (1987).

54 Brennan, M.; Davison, P.F.; Paulus, H.: Preparation of bispecific antibodies by chemical recombination of monoclonal immunoglobulin GI fragments. Science 229: 81–83 (1985).

55 Clark, M.R.; Waldmann, H.: T-cell killing of target cells induced by hybrid antibodies: comparison of two bispecific monoclonal antibodies. J. natn. Cancer Inst. 79: 1393–1401 (1987).

56 Scott, C.F.; Blattler, W.A.; Lambert, J.M.; Kalish, R.S.; Morimoto, C.; Schlossman, S.F.: Requirements for the construction of antibody heterodimers for the direction of lysis of tumors by human T cells. J. clin. Invest. 81: 1427–1433 (1988).

57 Rosenberg, S.A.: Immunotherapy of cancer using interleukin 2: current status and future prospects. Immunol. Today 9: 58–62 (1988).

58 Goldmacher, V.S.; Scott, C.F.; Lambert, J.M.; McIntyre, G.D.; Blattler, W.A.; Collinson, A.R.; Stewart, J.K.; Chong, L.D.; Cook, S.; Slayter, H.S.; Beaumont, E.; Watkins, S.: Cytotoxicity of gelonin and its conjugates with antibodies is determined by the extent of their endocytosis (submitted, 1988).

59 Glennie, M.J.; Brennand, D.M.; Bryden, F.; McBride, H.M.; Stirpe, F.; Worth, A.T.; Stevenson, G.T.: Bispecific F(ab')₂ antibody for the delivery of saporin in the treatment of lymphoma. J. Immun. 141: 3662–3670 (1988).

60 Lamm, M.E.; Boyse, E.A.; Old, L.J.; Lisowska-Bernstein, B.; Stockert, E.: Modulation of TL (thymus-leukemia) antigens by Fab-fragments of TL antibody. J. Immun. 101: 99–103 (1968).

61 Lanzavecchia, A.: Antigen-specific interaction between T and B cells. Nature, Lond. 314: 537–539 (1985).

62 Grey, H.M.; Chesnut, R.: Antigen processing and presentation to T cells. Immunol. Today 6: 101–106 (1985).

63 Germain, R.: Antigen processing and CD4⁺ T cell depletion in AIDS. Cell 54: 441–444 (1988).

64 Tite, J.P.; Powell, M.B.; Ruddle, N.H.: Protein-antigen specific 1a-restricted cytolytic T cells: analysis of frequency, target cell susceptibility, and mechanism of cytolysis. J. Immun. 135: 25–33 (1985).

65 Lukacher, A.E.; Morrison, L.A.; Braciale, V.L.; Malissew, B.; Braciale, T.J.: Expression of specific cytolitic activity by H-21 region-restricted, influenza virus-specific T lymphocyte clones. J. exp. Med. 162: 171–187 (1985).

66 Nakamura, M.; Ross, D.G.; Briner, T.J.; Gefter, M.L.: Cytolytic activity of antigen-specific T cells with helper phenotype. J. Immun. *136:* 44–47 (1986).

67 Ju, S.T.; DeKruyff, R.H.; Dorf, M.E.: Inducer T-cell-mediated killing of antigen-presenting cells. Cell. Immunol. *101:* 613–624 (1986).

68 Rock, K.L.; Benacerraf, B.; Abbas, A.K.: Antigen presentation by hapten-specific B lymphocytes. I. Role of surface immunoglobulin receptors. J. exp. Med. *160:* 1102–1113 (1984).

69 Ochi, A.; Worton, K.S.; Woods, G.; Gravelle, M.; Kitagami, K.: A novel strategy for immunotherapy using antibody-coupled carriers to focus cytotoxic T helper cells. Eur. J. Immunol. *17:* 1645–1648 (1987).

70 Lanzavecchia, A.; Abrignani, S.; Scheidegger, D.; Obrist, R.; Dorken, B.; Molden-hauer, G.: Antibodies as antigens. Use of mouse monoclonal antibodies to focus human T cells against selected targets. J. exp. Med. *167:* 345–352 (1988).

71 Lachmann, P.J.; Strangeways, L.; Vyakarnam, A.; Evan, G.: Raising antibodies by coupling peptides to PPD and immunizing BCG-sensitized animals; in Synthetic peptides as antigens. Ciba Foundation Symp. 119, pp. 25–57 (Wiley, Chichester 1986).

72 Townsend, A.R.; Rothbard, J.; Gotch, F.M.; Bahadur, G.; Wraith, D.; McMichael, A.J.: The epitopes of influenza nucleoprotein recognized by cytotoxic T lymphocytes can be defined with short synthetic peptides. Cell *44:* 959–968 (1986).

73 Lynch, R.G.; Rohrer, J.W.; Odermatt, B.; Gebel, H.M.; Autry, J.R.; Hoover, R.G.: Immunoregulation of murine myeloma cell growth and differentiation. A mono-clonal model of B cell differentiation. Immunol. Rev. *48:* 45–80 (1979).

74 Mellstedt, H.; Pettersson, D.; Holm, G.: Monoclonal B-lymphocytes in peripheral blood of patients with plasma cell myeloma: relation to activity of the disease. Scand. J. Haematol. *16:* 112–120 (1976).

75 Eisen, H.N.; Sakato, N.; Hall, S.J.: Myeloma proteins as tumor-specific antigens. Transplant. Proc. *VII:* 209–214 (1975).

76 Stevenson, F.K.; Gregg, E.O.; Smith, J.L.; Stevenson, G.T.: Secretion of immuno-globulin by neoplastic B lymphocytes from lymph nodes of patients with lymphoma. Br. J. Cancer *50:* 579–586 (1984).

77 Thielemans, K.; Maloney, D.G.; Meeker, T.; Fugimoto, J.; Doss, C.; Warnke, R.A.; Bindl, J.; Gralow, J.; Miller, R.A.; Levy, R.: Strategies for production of monoclonal anti-idiotype antibodies against human B cell lymphomas. J. Immun. *133:* 495–501 (1984).

78 Stevenson, F.K.; Gordon, J.: Immunization with idiotypic immunoglobulin protects against development of B lymphocyte leukemia, but emerging tumor cells can evade antibody attack by modulation. J. Immun. *130:* 970–973 (1983).

79 George, A.J.T.; Tutt, A.L.; Stevenson, F.K.: Anti-idiotypic mechanisms involved in suppression of a mouse B cell lymphoma, BCL_1. J. Immun. *138:* 628–634 (1987).

80 Campbell, M.J.; Carroll, W.; Kou, S.; Thielemans, K.; Rothbard, J.B.; Levy, S.; Levy, R.: Idiotype vaccination against murine B cell lymphoma. Humoral and cellular responses elicited by tumor-derived immunoglobulin H and its molecular subunits. J. Immun. *139:* 2825–2833 (1987).

81 Slavin, S.; Strober, S.: Spontaneous murine B cell leukemia. Nature, Lond. *272:* 624–626 (1977).

82 Vitetta, E.S.; Krolick, K.A.; Uhr, J.W.: Neoplastic B cells as targets for antibody-ricin A chain immunotoxins. Immunol. Rev. *62:* 159–183 (1982).

83 Krolick, K.A.; Isakson, P.C.; Uhr, J.W.; Vitetta, E.S.: BCL$_1$, a murine model for chronic lymphocytic leukemia: use of the surface immunoglobulin idiotype for the detection and treatment of tumor. Immunol. Rev. 48: 81–106 (1979).

84 Tutt, A.L.; Stevenson, F.K.; Slavin, S.; Stevenson, G.T.: Secretion of idiotypic IgM by the mouse B-cell leukaemia (BCL$_1$) occurs spontaneously in vitro and in vivo. Immunology 55: 59–63 (1985).

85 George, A.J.T.; Folkard, S.G.; Hamblin, T.J.; Stevenson, F.K.: Idiotypic vaccination as a treatment for a B cell lymphoma. J. Immun. 141: 2168–2174 (1988).

86 Greenberg, P.D.; Cheever, M.A.; Fefer, A.: Prerequisites for successful adaptive immunotherapy: nature of effector cells and role of H-2 restriction; in Fefer, Goldstein, The potential role of T cells in cancer therapy, pp. 31–50 (Raven Press, New York 1982).

87 Sakato, N.; Hall, S.H.; Eisen, H.N.: Suppression of MOPC-167 growth in vivo by immunization against the idiotype of the MOPC-167 myeloma protein. Microbiol. Immunol. 23: 927–931 (1979).

88 Bridges, S.H.: Participation of the humoral immune system in the myeloma-specific transplantation resistance. J. Immun. 121: 479–483 (1978).

89 Frikke, M.J.; Bridges, S.H.; Lynch, R.G.: Myeloma-specific antibodies: studies of their properties and their relationship to tumor immunity. J. Immun. 118: 2206–2212 (1977).

90 Freedman, P.M.; Autry, J.R.; Tokuda, S.; Williams, R.C., Jr.: Tumor immunity induced by preimmunization with BALB/c mouse myeloma protein. J. natn. Cancer Inst. 56: 735–740 (1976).

91 Kaminski, M.S.; Kitamura, K.; Maloney, D.G.; Campbell, M.J.; Levy, R.: Importance of antibody isotype in monoclonal anti-idiotype therapy of a murine B cell lymphoma. A study of hybridoma class switch variants. J. Immun. 136: 1123–1130 (1986).

92 Chen, Y.; Yakulis, V.; Heller, P.: Passive immunity to murine plasmacytoma by rabbit anti-idiotypic antibody to myeloma protein. Proc. Soc. exp. Biol. Med. 151: 121–125 (1976).

93 Stevenson, G.T.; Elliott, E.V.; Stevenson, F.K.: Idiotypic determinants on the surface immunoglobulin of neoplastic lymphocytes. A therapeutic target. Fed. Proc. 36: 2268–2271 (1977).

94 Milburn, G.L.; Parslow, T.G.; Goldenberg, C.; Granner, D.K.; Lynch, R.G.: Idiotype-specific T cell suppression of light chain in RNA expression in MODC-315 cells is accompanied by a posttranscriptional inhibition of heavy chain expression. J. mol. Cell Immunol. 1: 115–123 (1984).

95 Abbas, A.K.; Perry, L.L.; Bach, B.A.; Greene, H.L.: Idiotype-specific T cell immunity. I. Generation of effector and suppressor T lymphocytes reactive with myeloma idiotypic determinants. J. Immun. 124: 1160–1166 (1980).

96 Sakato. N.; Semma, H.; Eisen, H.N.; Azuma, T.: A small hypervariable segment in the variable domain of an immunoglobulin light chain stimulates formation of anti-idiotype suppressor T cells. Proc. natn. Acad. Sci. USA 79: 5396–5400 (1982).

97 Hannestad, K.; Kristoffersen, G.; Briand, J.P.: The T lymphocyte response to syngeneic λ2 light chain idiotopes. Significance of individual amino acids revealed by variant λ2 chains and idiotope-mimicking chemically synthesized peptides. Eur. J. Immunol. 16: 889–893 (1986).

98 Jorgensen, T.; Hannestad, K.: Specificity of T and B lymphocytes for myeloma protein 315. Eur. J. Immunol. 7: 426–431 (1977).

99 Jorgensen, T.; Hannestad, K.: H-2-linked genes control immune response to V-domains of myeloma protein 315. Nature, Lond. *288:* 396–397 (1980).

100 Jorgensen, T.; Ganderneck, G.; Hannestad, K.: Immunization with the light chain and the V_L domain of the isologous myeloma protein 315 inhibits growth of mouse plasmacytoma MOPC 315. Scand. J. Immunol. *11:* 29–35 (1980).

101 Bogen, B.; Malissen, B.; Haas, W.: Idiotope-specific T cell clones that recognize syngeneic immunoglobulin fragments in the context of class II molecules. Eur. J. Immunol. *16:* 1273–1278 (1986).

102 Waters, S.J.; Bona, C.A.: Characterization of a T-cell clone recognizing idiotypes as tumor-associated antigens. Cell. Immunol. *111:* 87–93 (1988).

103 Ghosh, S.K.; Bankert, R.B.: Generation of heavy chain-loss mutants in a B cell hybrid mediated by syngeneic idiotype-specific spleen cells. J. Immun. *133:* 1677–1682 (1984).

104 Ghosh, S.K.; Wong, J.; Bankert, R.B.: Idiotype-specific T lymphocytes responsible for the selection of somatic variants of a B cell hybrid. J. Immun. *138:* 2230–2235 (1987).

105 Wheelock, E.F.; Robinson, M.K.: Biology of disease. Endogenous control of the neoplastic process. Lab. Invest. *48:* 120–139 (1983).

106 Krolick, K.A.; Uhr, J.W.; Slavin, S.; Vitetta, E.S.: In vivo therapy of a murine B cell tumor (BCL_1) using antibody-ricin A chain immunotoxins. J. exp. Med. *155:* 1797–1809 (1982).

107 Starnes, C.O.; Carroll, W.L.; Campbell, M.J.; Houston, L.L.; Apell, G.; Levy, R.: Heterogeneity of a murine B cell lymphoma. Isolation and characterization of idiotype variants. J. Immun. *141:* 333–339 (1988).

108 Krikorian, J.G.; Portlock, C.S.; Cooney, D.P.; Rosenberg, S.A.: Spontaneous regression of non-Hodgkin's lymphoma. A report of nine cases. Cancer *46:* 2093–2099 (1980).

Freda K. Stevenson, D. Phil., Lymphoma Research Unit, Tenovus Research Laboratory, General Hospital, Southampton, S09 4XY (UK)

Carson DA, Chen PP, Kipps TJ (eds): Idiotypes in Biology and Medicine.
Chem Immunol. Basel, Karger, 1990, vol 48, pp 167–185

Immunoglobulin Idiotypes in Human B Cell Neoplasia

Implications for Pathogenesis and Therapy[1]

Thomas J. Kipps

Department of Molecular and Experimental Medicine, Scripps Clinic and Research Foundation, La Jolla, Calif., USA

There is considerable interest in immunotherapy of human malignancy [1, 2]. This is evident particularly since the advent of monoclonal antibody (mAb) technology, allowing for the generation of virtually unlimited amounts of antibody of desired binding activity [3]. The introduction of genetically engineered antibodies having both specificity for a tumor antigen and enhanced capacity for directing specific antitumor cytotoxicity has increased the likelihood that mAbs may act effectively as 'magic bullets' in the treatment of neoplastic disease [Stevenson et al., pp. 126–166]. Finally, through elucidation of the mechanics of immune recognition and tolerance, effective active immunotherapy of human malignancy may become feasible. Identification and characterization of 'tumor-specific' surface antigens should allow us to generate mAb reactive with, and synthetic antigens corresponding to, exposed structural determinants that may be useful in both passive and active immunotherapy.

Immunotherapy of B Cell Malignancy

Human B cell malignancy should be amenable to both forms of immunotherapy. The variable region of surface immunoglobulin (sIg) expressed by

[1] Research reviewed in this report supported in part by Grants No. AR38475, AR33489, AG04100, and RR00833 from the National Institutes of Health. Dr. Kipps is a Scholar of the Leukemia Society of America, funded in part by the Scott Helping Hand Fund, and recipient of an Investigator Award from the Arthritis Foundation. This is publication No. 5773-BCR from the Research Institute of Scripps Clinic.

malignant cells may possess unique idiotypic specificities and subgroup determinants that are clonally distributed. As such, the variable region of sIg expressed by a clone of malignant B cells constitutes a truly tumor-specific surface marker [4–8]. Development in our knowledge of immunoglobulin gene expression in B lymphoid neoplasia may allow us to devise new strategies for effective immunotherapy.

Immunoglobulin Variable Region Structure

The antibody variable region is formed by the juxtaposition of two polypeptide immunoglobulin chains encoded by genes located on different chromosomes [9–11]. Each chain is encoded by discontinuous genetic elements that rearrange to form novel immunoglobulin genes during B cell ontogeny [12–14]. In the embryonic kappa-light chain gene complex, for example, there are many kappa-V genes (V_K) arranged in tandem. Through rearrangement, one V_K is juxtaposed with one of five joining segments (J_K) to form a VJ complex that encodes the variable region of the kappa-light chain [15–17]. The heavy chain complex is arranged similarly except that it has additional genetic elements, named the diversity segments (D), positioned between the V_H genes and six functional J_H genes [18–20]. At least one D segment is juxtaposed with the single J_H before rearranging with a V_H gene to form a VDJ complex which encodes the variable portion of the antibody heavy chain [21, 22].

Comparisons of the primary amino acid sequences of many different antibody variable regions reveals four regions of limited amino acid sequence diversity, designated the framework regions [23]. Examination of the first three variable region frameworks reveals that the human heavy and light chain variable regions may be classified into subgroups. Each variable region subgroup has characteristic framework sequences that serve to distinguish it from other variable region subgroups. Initially, human heavy chains were divided into three subgroups, while kappa- and lambda-light chains were divided into four and six subgroups, respectively.

Recently, variable region amino acid subgroup homologies have been found to extend to the nucleic acid sequence level [24–32], confirming the anticipation that immunoglobulin subgroups defined families of highly related antibody variable region genes (V genes). Cloned V genes with deduced amino acid sequences belonging to a given subgroup generally share greater than 80% nucleic acid sequence homology. Recent exceptions to this generalization have resulted in the identification of a novel heavy chain variable gene subgroup, subgroup 4 [33, 34]. The deduced amino acid sequences for heavy chain V genes (v_H genes) of this subgroup share homology with members of protein subgroup 2. However, at the nucleic acid level, these genes are less than 70% homologous to V_H genes previously reported to represent the $V_H 2$ gene family. Thus, these V_H genes are reasoned members of a novel V_H gene family. Recent isolation of additional V_H genes has revealed the existence of two additional V_H gene subgroups not previously identified at the amino acid level, designated $V_H 5$ and $V_H 6$ [32, 35, 36]. V_H genes of the $V_H 5$ subgroup are most related to members of the $V_H 1$ family, and the apparently single-copy $V_H 6$ gene is most related to V_H genes of the $V_H 4$ subgroup. Unlike the noted protein sequence homology between $V_H 2$ and $V_H 4$, however, the deduced amino acid framework sequences of either $V_H 5$ or $V_H 6$ are subgroup specific.

Differences in the primary amino acid sequences between the various immunoglobulin subgroups result in structural differences in the antibody variable region that can be detected serologically [37–41]. Crystallographic data of isolated light and heavy chain variable regions demonstrate that the first framework region of either chain forms a beta-bend on the external surface of the molecule [42–46]. As such, amino acid differences noted between the different variable region subgroups should be amenable to immune recognition. Using isolated light chains as immunogens, and carefully absorbed rabbit antisera, serologic reagents with subgroup specificity have been derived [41]. Furthermore, a few mAb generated against intact immunoglobulin molecules fortuitously have been found to have subgroup specificity [47, 48]. Recently, antisera highly specific for each of the kappa-variable region subgroups [49], or for each of V_H subgroups 1 to 3 [50], have been generated using synthetic peptides corresponding to subgroup-specific primary amino acid sequences in the first framework region of the kappa-light chain V region or heavy chain V region, respectively. Thus, the epitope(s) within the first framework may serve to distinguish clones of sIg bearing B cells with respect to expressed variable region subgroup.

Positioned between the framework regions are three segments of extreme hypervariability in both light and heavy chain sequences [23]. The third hypervariable region is generated in part by the recombinatorial process joining the antibody light chain V gene with the J segment, in the case of the light chain, or the V_H gene with the somatically generated DJ segment of the antibody heavy chain [12, 15, 18–20]. The diversity of the first and second hypervariable regions partly reflects germline DNA-encoded differences between disparate antibody V genes, a diversity often noted even between V genes of the same subgroup [24–32]. Somatic events subsequent to V gene rearrangement, however, have been found to play an important role in increasing the diversity noted within these regions (discussed below). Affinity labeling and crystallographic experiments have substantiated earlier contentions that the hypervariable regions on both chains fold together to form the antigen-combining site [42–46]. Hence, these regions of hypervariability are designated the complementarity-determining regions (CDRs) [23]. These regions may form determinants of unique specificity that can be recognized by anti-idiotypic antibodies.

Idiotype Heterogeneity

Clinical trials testing the efficacy of monoclonal anti-idiotypic antibodies in the treatment of human B cell lymphomas have yielded mixed results [1, 51–54]. Despite the initial success reported with 1 patient [51], subsequent patients that received tailor-made anti-idiotypic antibodies have failed to achieve complete and/or long-lasting partial remissions. Of note, however, is the fairly high response rate noted in some of these studies. In one study, 9 of the 13 patients (70%) with chemotherapy-refractory disease had objective tumor responses to administered monoclonal anti-idiotypic antibody [53, 55]. Although 8 of these patients relapsed within 1–12 months, 5 of these 8 relapsing patients had recurrent lymphomas that were nonreactive to the original anti-idiotypic antibodies used in therapy. Thus, although not completely effective in eliminating the disease, the administered monoclonal anti-idiotypic antibodies apparently selected against the growth of idiotype-bearing cells.

Idiotype-negative variants apparently arise through somatic mutation of the immunoglobulin genes expressed by these lymphomas. Escaping tumor populations generally express sIg at amounts comparable to that of the original tumor population [55–57]. Molecular analyses of the expressed immunoglobulin genes of parent and variant populations reveal the VD and DJ junctions of the antibody heavy chain variable region and the VJ junction of the antibody light chain are conserved, indicating that the tumor populations of any one patient are clonally related. Furthermore, lymphoma subpopulations also are noted to share chromosomal translocations that have identical molecular breakpoints, confirming the clonal origin of both parent and idiotype-negative variant populations [58].

Nucleic acid sequence analyses of the immunoglobulin V genes ex-pressed by individual cells of such clonally related lymphoma populations reveal extensive V gene heterogeneity. In fact, no two hybridomas generated from such lymphomas expressed identical heavy or light chain V genes [55, 59]. Nucleic acid base differences were found concentrated in the V gene, but also were noted in the 5′ untranslated region. Overall, the pattern of substitutions seen suggests that the process(es) of somatic hypermutation noted in V genes expressed during secondary immune responses is operating in these lymphomas [60, 61].

Of particular importance, the amino acid replacement mutations are nonrandomly distributed within the variable region [55]. Amino acid repla-cement mutations are noted to be much less frequent in the framework regions than would be anticipated if the nucleic acid substitutions were occurring randomly. In contrast, extensive amino acid substitutions are noted in the CDR, particularly CDR2. Moreover, a high percentage of the nucleic acid mutations observed in CDR2 are nonconservative.

The mechanism(s) responsible for the nonstochastic distribution of non-conservative nucleic acid substitutions in the V genes expressed by these lymphomas is unknown. To be sure, this mechanism(s) apparently operates independent of the selection imposed by monoclonal anti-idiotypic antibodies, as idiotypic heterogeneity is noted in such lymphomas even prior to passive immunotherapy [62, 63]. Perhaps selective forces within the tumor-bearing host act to reduce the growth advantage of malignant cells expressing V genes with mutations causing amino acid changes within the framework regions. Such selection may be negative, operating to eliminate cells expressing permuted variable region frameworks, or positive, providing growth advantage only to those lymphoma cells that express sIg without amino acid substitutions in critical framework regions that furnish the scaffolding for the antigen-combining site. Alternatively, nucleic acid substitutions resulting in amino acid replacements in the framework regions may occur infrequently because of the mechanics of somatic hypermutation. Such a process may involve gene conversion between highly related V genes belonging to similar or identical V gene subgroups that have disparate CDRs but similar or identical variable region frameworks.

Cross-Reactive Idiotypes

Despite the enormous potential for diversity in immunoglobulin V gene expression and genetic polymorphisms, antibodies produced by B cell malignancies of unrelated persons may share common idiotypic determinants. Initially defined using absorbed heterologous antisera [64], and then more recently using murine mAbs [48, 65, 66], these common idiotopes, designated cross-reactive idiotopes (CRIs), were identified initially on IgM autoantibodies, such as rheumatoid factors. That such CRIs were not merely the tertiary reflections of a shared binding activity, however, were indicated by protein-sequence data demonstrating that the light or heavy chain variable regions of CRI-bearing immunoglobulins may have conserved primary structure [67–72]. Thus, such CRIs resemble more the CRIs of antibodies produced in inbred mice that are encoded by antibody V genes present in the germline-DNA.

Certain human B cell malignancies frequently express antibodies bearing major CRIs. In a study of over 30 patients with chronic lymphocytic leukemia (CLL), 5 of 20 (25%) patients with kappa-light-chain-expressing CLL had malignant cells that expressed a CRI defined by reactivity with a mAb, designated 17.109 [73, 74]. This antibody, prepared against an RF paraprotein, recognizes a kappa-light-chain-associated CRI present on a high proportion of human IgM RF paraproteins isolated from patients with Waldenstrom's macroglobulinemia [65, 75, 76]. Furthermore, greater than 20% (8/34) of both kappa- and lambda-light-chain-expressing CLL were found to react with G6 [77], an mAb specific for an Ig heavy-chain-associated CRI present on several RF paraproteins [66]. Interestingly, 40% (2/5) of the CLL cases with leukemic cells reactive with 17.109 also reacted with G6, reflecting a biased co-expression of these CRIs.

Multiparameter flow cytometric analyses indicated that CRI expression by leukemic cells is not qualitatively heterogeneous [78]. Dual immunofluorescence studies using fluorescein-labeled antibodies specific for the antibody constant region and phycoerythrin-conjugated anti-cross-reactive idiotype antibodies demonstrated that the relative staining intensities of anti-cross-reactive idiotype mAbs correlated directly with the relative number of expressed sIg molecules. Furthermore, CRI-negative but sIg-positive leukemic cells were not detected in any leukemic cell population studied. Moreover, differences in the relative staining intensities of our anti-cross-reactive idiotype on leukemic cell populations from different patients were found secondary to differences in relative levels of expressed sIg. These data demonstrate that different levels of CRI expression by cells within or between leukemic populations are not secondary to qualitative structural differences in the cross-reactive idiotype, but rather secondary to the level of sIg expressed by the leukemic cells. These data argue that, unlike the lymphomas discussed earlier, antibody gene expression in CLL is stable.

Molecular Basis for Cross-Reactive Idiotype Expression

In order to examine the molecular basis for the 17.109-cross-reactive idiotype expression in CLL, we isolated and sequenced the kappa variable region genes from unrelated CLL patients with 17.109-reactive lymphocytes [78]. Analyses of multiple independent cDNA clones did not reveal any sequence heterogeneity between the kappa V genes (V_k genes) expressed within a CLL population from any one patient. Furthermore, 17.109-reactive leukemic cells from unrelated patients express nearly identical V_k genes, these belonging to the V_kIIIb sub-subgroup. Finally, the sequences of the V_k genes expressed by 17.109-reactive leukemic cells share greater than 99% nucleic acid sequence identity to a germline V_kIII gene isolated from placental DNA, designed *Humkv325* [79]. Thus, the 17.109-cross-reactive idiotype in CLL apparently is secondary to the expression of a highly conserved kappa-variable gene with little or no somatic mutation.

The high frequency expression of the 17.109-cross-reactive idiotype in CLL indicates that the usage of variable region genes in this B cell malignancy is nonrandom. Estimates of the number of distinct V_k genes range from 25 to 75 [27–30]. To date, over 35 V_k genes have been distinguished [27–30, 80, 81]. Of these, 8 belong to the V_kIII subgroup [80, 81]. Only one of these, *Humkv325*, has nucleic acid sequence homology with the V_k gene expressed by the 17.109-cross-reactive idiotype bearing leukemic cells. Moreover, only *Humkv325* can encode the kappa light chain paraproteins that are recognized by 17.109 without sequence permutation.

Similarly, examination of the molecular basis for the G6-cross-reactive idiotype in CLL revealed the G6 idiotope(s) to be a serologic marker for expression of a conserved V_H gene of the V_H1 subgroup [82]. Amino acid sequence data of Waldenstrom's RF paraproteins demonstrated that G6-reactive IgM RF share considerable sequence homology in the first, second and fourth frameworks of the heavy chain variable region [83]. From these data, it had been deduced that the heavy chain variable regions of G6-reactive RF were encoded by V_H gene(s) of the V_H1 subgroup, a relatively short D segment, and the J_H4 gene segment. Nucleic acid sequence analyses revealed G6-reactive leukemic cells from unrelated CLL patients express nearly identical V_H1 genes that share greater than 99% nucleic acid sequence homology [82]. Despite expressing near identical V_H genes, however, G6-reactive leukemic cells may express markedly different D segments and utilize J_H6 or J_H4 gene segments. Comparisons of the deduced amino acid sequences of G6-reactive CLL and that of G6-negative antibody heavy chains encoded by

V_H1 genes suggests that the G6-CRI in CLL is relatively resilient to substitutions within CDR3, but affected by permutations within CDR1 and CDR2. Together these data argue that the G6-CRI in CLL is a serologic marker for a conserved V_H1 gene expressed with little or no somatic diversification.

That a relatively high precentage of CLL express the G6 or 17.109 cross-reactive idiotype raises the possibility that the variable region protein structures recognized by these antibodies actually may affect leukemogenesis indirectly. Both are commonly found on IgM autoantibodies, particularly RF [66, 75, 76]. Furthermore, co-expression of both cross-reactive idiotypes invariably have been detected only on IgM antibodies with RF activity [50]. The sIg of a high proportion of CLL have been reported to have such RF activity [74, 84]. Perhaps B lymphocytes with such self-reactive sIg may be stimulated to divide constitutively, thereby increasing the likelihood for chance transformation. Autoreactive sIg also may serve to focus a transforming agent onto the cell, for example, by binding a leukemogenic virus or antigen-antibody complexes containing such a transforming agent [85]. In this light, it is perhaps noteworthy that a recently elucidated amino acid sequence of the kappa-light chain variable region from a human anti-cyto-megalovirus IgG_k shares extensive homology with the deduced amino acid sequence of 17.109-reactive CLL B cells, and probably is encoded by the same V_k gene [86].

Alternatively, the V genes encoding these CRIs may be used repeatedly by the normal B cell subpopulation that may be subject to malignant transformation in CLL. CLL is a malignancy of cells that co-express B cell-specific surface antigens and CD5 (Leu 1, OKT1), a 67-kdalton surface protein present on peripheral T cells [87–91]. The physiologic counterpart to such cells is the CD5 B cell [92]. These cells constitute a small subpopulation of human B lymphocytes in lymphoid organs and peripheral blood of normal adults [93–96]. Such CD5 B lymphocytes (commonly termed 'Leu 1 B cells') are speculated to have functional properties similar to murine B cells expressing the mouse CD5 homolog, Ly-1 [95, 97–99]. These latter cells may spontaneously secrete IgM autoantibodies [97] and amplify production of specific antibodies with restricted idiotypes through B-B cell interaction in vitro [100–103]. Recently, human CD5 B cells have also been found to have possible immunoregulatory capacities [104, 105], and to be enriched in cells producing IgM autoantibodies [106, 107]. The latter suggests that the expressed antibody repertoire of human CD5 B cells may be distinct from that of B lymphocytes that do not express the CD5 surface antigen.

The apparent restriction in the repertoire of V genes epxressed in CLL may in part reflect a genetically programmed restriction in the expression of antibody V genes by the CD5 B cell. Consistent with this notion, the V_H1 gene utilized by G6-reactive CLL is homologous with 51p1, a V_H1 gene expressed during early B cell ontogeny. This is remarkable considering that the set of V_H genes that are expressed during early fetal development is highly restricted [36]. Of the V_H genes isolated from the fetal liver library, one accounted for the expression of over 20% (3/14) of the heavy chain sequences while three others each accounted for 14% (2/14) of the sequences. Statistical analyses of these data infer that the total size of the fetal V_H repertoire is between 9 and 39 elements. Early restriction in fetal V gene expression is noted prior to development of mature sIg-expressing B cells and, hence, may be programmed genetically [36]. Homology between the V_H gene expressed by G6-reactive CLL and a V_H gene frequently utilized in the highly restricted fetal repertoire suggests that the set of V genes expressed in CLL may be comparable to that utilized during early B cell development. Such a hypothesis is tenable considering that the physiologic counterpart to CLL, the CD5 B cell, constitutes the predominant B cell subpopulation in human fetal spleen and liver, presumably when the repertoire of expressed V genes is still restricted [108, 109].

Should the mechanism(s) that restricts V gene expression during B cell ontogeny also restrict V gene expression in CLL, then we would predict that the V genes encoding the major CLL-associated CRIs are rearranged more often than they are expressed. Consistent with this are preliminary data indicating that the *Humkv325* V_k gene encoding the 17.109-cross-reactive idiotype is rearranged abortively in many CLL expressing lambda-light chains [110]. The mechanism(s) accounting for this is not known. One hypothesis is that the relative order of V genes positioned along the chromosomes may affect their relative expression frequencies, as has been demonstrated in the mouse [111–113]. However, mapping studies of the human immunoglobulin kappa-light chain locus demonstrates that many functional V_k genes are located between the J_k locus and *Humkv325* [114]. Thus, frequent abortive rearrangements of the *Humkv325* in CLL cannot be explained simply by chromosomal order. In this regard, the rearrangement of *Humkv325* in CLL may be similar to that of a recently identified V_H5 gene, designated V_H251 [115]. Although not the most proximal V_H gene to the D and J regions, this gene was found to be rearranged with the DJ segment in greater than 20% of over 30 patient studied [115].

Mechanism(s) providing for preferential V gene rearrangement alone, however, may not account for the frequent expression of autoantibody cross-reactive idiotype in CLL. As noted above, approximately 40% of the CLL that are 17.109-cross-reactive idiotype positive also express the G6-cross-reactive idiotype. This indicates a biased co-expression of *Humkv325* with the V_H1 gene(s) encoding the G6-cross-reactive idiotype. As such, both preferential rearrangement and selected co-expression of particular antibody V genes may occur in CLL.

Expression of CRIs in Other B Cell Malignancies

We also examined solid-tissue non-Hodgkin's lymphomas (NHL) to determine the relative incidence of the 17.109 or G6 cross-reactive idiotypes. Although cross-reactive idiotypes have been detected on NHL from unrelated patients [116], expression of the autoantibody-associated CRIs is rare in NHL of follicular center cell origin [77]. These NHL do not express the CD5 surface antigen and hence may be derived from a B cell lineage(s) or stage(s) of differentiation distinct from that of CLL. On the other hand, B cell NHL that frequently co-express CD5, such as small lymphocytic lymphoma [117–122], express these CRIs at frequencies comparable to that noted in CLL [123]. These studies reveal a fundamental distinction between CD5-positive and CD5-negative human B malignancies with respect to the expression of autoantibody-associated CRIs. The data support the notion that these B cell malignancies differ in their utilization and/or somatic diversification of expressed immunoglobulin V genes.

Support for the notion that there exists a distinction between CD5-positive and CD5-negative B cell malignancies in their respective rates of somatic hypermutation comes from analyses of the relative expression frequencies of variable region framework determinants. Somatic mutation in the expressed antibody V gene may permute and distort antigenic determinants that form the CRIs. However, as mentioned above, variable region framework determinants are relatively resilient to the process of somatic hypermutation. For our studies, we stained cells with an mAb specific for V_kIIIb kappa-light framework determinants [47]. Of our panel of CLL patients, we noted that the anti-V_kIIIb antibody reacts exclusively with cells bearing the 17.109-cross-reactive idiotype, suggesting that the *Humkv325* gene is the predominant V_kIIIb gene expressed in this malignancy. In contrast, only one of three CD5-negative expressing NHL found reactive with the V_kIIIb expressed the 17.109-cross-reactive idiotpye. However, the proportion of kappa-light-chain expressing CD5-negative NHL that react with the mAb is comparable to the frequencies with which this mAb reacts with kappa-light chain expressing CLL or CD5-positive NHL. These results are consistent with the notion that the relatively low expression frequencies of cross-reactive idiotypes by CD5-negative NHL may be related in part to somatic diversification of the same V genes expressed in CD5 B cell malignancies.

Relevance to Immunotherapy

Identification of additional CRIs may afford a partial answer to the problems associated with immunotherapy. The necessity to generate idiotype-specific mAbs against each patient's malignant clone makes this form of therapy extremely costly and time consuming [124]. Clinical studies comparing the role of immunoglobulin isotype, mode of mAb delivery, utility of antibody-toxin conjugates and the relative advantages of single versus multiple mAb therapy, have been confounded by the need to tailor a unique reagent for each patient studied. The recognition of conserved CRIs expressed by malignant B lymphocytes may permit the production of batteries of mAb reagents suitable for the early diagnosis and possible future immunotherapy of a large number of patients with CD5 B cell malignancies.

Already we have discerned an apparent major distinction between CD5 B malignancies and CD5-negative B cell tumors with respect to the biology of immunoglobulin gene expression. Should we better define these distinctions with additional molecular and biochemical studies, we may elucidate differences in immunoglobulin V gene expression that are important in understanding disease pathogenesis and in developing more effective means for sIg-directed immunotherapy.

References

1 Stevenson, G.T.: The prospects for treating cancer with antibody. Sci. Prog. *70:* 505–519 (1986).
2 Reisfeld, R.A.; Cheresh, D.A.: Human tumor antigens. Adv. Immunol. *40:* 323–327 (1987).
3 Kohler, G.; Milstein, C.: Derivation of specific antibody-producing tissue culture and tumor lines by cell fusion. Eur. J. Immunol. *6:* 511–519 (1976).
4 Lynch, R.G.; Graff, R.J.; Sirisinha, S.; Simms, E.S.; Eisen, H.N.: Myeloma proteins as tumor-specific transplantation antigens. Proc. natn. Acad. Sci. USA *69:* 1540–1544 (1972).

5 Schroer, K.R.; Briles, D.E.; Van Boxel, J.A.; Davie, J.M.: Idiotypic uniformity of cell surface immunoglobulin in chronic lymphocytic leukemia. Evidence for monoclonal proliferation. J. exp. Med. *140:* 1416–1420 (1974).

6 Stevenson, G.T.; Stevenson, F.K.: Antibody to a molecularly-defined antigen confined to a tumour cell surface. Nature, Lond. *254:* 714–716 (1975).

7 Stevenson, G.T.; Elliott, E.V.; Stevenson, F.K.: Idiotypic determinants on the surface immunoglobulin of neoplastic lymphocytes. A therapeutic target. Fed. Proc. *36:* 2268–2271 (1977).

8 Haughton, G.; Lanier, L.L.; Babcock, G.F.; Lynes, M.A.: Antigen-induced murine B cell lymphomas. II. Exploitation of the surface idiotype as tumor specific antigen. J. Immun. *121:* 2358–2362 (1978).

9 Malcolm, S.; Barton, P.; Murphy, C.; Ferguson-Smith, M.A.; Bentley, D.L.; Rabbitts, T.H.: Localization of human immunoglobulin kappa light chain variable region genes to the short arm of chromosome 2 by in situ hybridization. Proc. natn. Acad. Sci. USA *79:* 4957–4961 (1982).

10 McBride, O.W.; Hieter, P.A.; Hollis, G.F.; Swan, D.; Otey, M.C.; Leder, P.: Chromosomal location of human kappa and lambda immunoglobulin light chain constant region genes. J. exp. Med. *155:* 1480–1490 (1982).

11 Kirsch, I.R.; Morton, C.C.; Nakahara, K.; Leder, P.: Human immunoglobulin heavy chain gene map to a region of translocations in malignant B lymphocytes. Science *216:* 301–303 (1982).

12 Tonegawa, S.: Somatic generation of antibody diversity. Nature, Lond. *302:* 575–581 (1983).

13 Seidman, J.G.; Leder, P.: The arrangement and rearrangement of antibody genes. Nature, Lond. *276:* 790–795 (1978).

14 Seidman, J.G.; Leder, A.; Nau, M.; Norman, B.; Leder, P.: Antibody diversity. Science *202:* 11–17 (1978).

15 Brack, C.; Hirama, M.; Lenhard-Schuller, R.; Tonegawa, S.: A complete immunoglobulin gene is created by somatic recombination. Cell *15:* 1–14 (1978).

16 Seidman, J.G.; Nau, M.M.; Norman, B.; Kwan, S.P.; Scharff, M.; Leder, P.: Immunoglobulin V/J recombination is accompanied by deletion of joining site and variable region segments. Proc. natn. Acad. Sci. USA *77:* 6022–6026 (1980).

17 Hieter, P.A.; Max, E.E.; Seidman, J.G.; Maizel, J.V., Jr.; Leder, P.: Cloned human and mouse kappa immunoglobulin constant and J region genes conserve homology in functional segments. Cell *22:* 197–207 (1980).

18 Sakano, H.; Kurosawa, Y.; Weigert, M.; Tonegawa, S.: Identification and nucleotide sequence of a diversity DNA segment (D) of immunoglobulin heavy-chain genes. Nature, Lond. *290:* 562–565 (1981).

19 Siebenlist, U.; Ravetch, J.V.; Korsmeyer, S.; Waldmann, T.; Leder, P.: Human immunoglobulin D segments encoded in tandem multigenic families. Nature, Lond. *294:* 631–635 (1981).

20 Early, P.; Huang, H.; Davis, M.; Calame, K.; Hood, L.: An immunoglobulin heavy chain variable region gene is generated from three segments of DNA: VH, D and JH. Cell *19:* 981–992 (1980).

21 Yancopoulos, G.D.; Alt, F.W.: Regulation of the assembly and expression of variable-region genes. A. Rev. Immunol. *4:* 339–368 (1986).

22 Reth, M.G.; Jackson, S.; Alt, F.W.: VHDJH formation and DJH replacement during

pre-B non-random usage of gene segments. Eur. molec. Biol. Org. J. *5:* 2131–2138 (1986).

23 Kabat, E.; Wu, T.T.; Reid-Miller, M.; Perry, H.M.; Gottesmann, K.S.: Sequences of proteins of immunological interest (US Government Printing Office, Bethesda, MD 1987).

24 Matthyssens, G.; Rabbitts, T.H.: Structure and multiplicity of genes for the human immunoglobulin heavy chain variable region. Proc. natn. Acad. Sci. USA *77:* 6561–6565 (1980).

25 Rechavi, G.; Ram, D.; Glazer, L.; Zakut, R.; Givol, D.: Evolutionary aspcts of immunoglobulin heavy chain variable region (VH) gene subgroups. Proc. natn. Acad. Sci. USA *80:* 855–859 (1983).

26 Takahashi, N.; Noma, T.; Honjo, T.: Rearranged immunoglobulin heavy chain variable region (VH) pseudogene that deletes the second complementarity-determining region. Proc. natn. Acad. Sci. USA *81:* 5194–5198 (1984).

27 Bentley, D.L.: Most kappa immunoglobulin mRNA in human lymphocytes is homologous to a small family of germ-line V genes. Nature, Lond. *307:* 77–80 (1984).

28 Klobeck, H.G.; Solomon, A.; Zachau, H.G.: Contribution of human V kappa II germ-line genes to light-chain diversity. Nature, Lond. *309:* 73–76 (1984).

29 Jaenichen, H.R.; Pech, M.; Lindenmaier, W.; Wildgruber, N.; Zachau, H.G.: Composite human VK genes and a model of their evolution. Nucl. Acids Res. *12:* 5249–5263 (1984).

30 Pech, M.; Zachau, H.G.: Immunoglobulin genes of different subgroups are interdigitated within the VK locus. Nucl. Acids Res. *12:* 9229–9236 (1984).

31 Kodaira, M.; Kinashi, T.; Umemura, I.; et al.: Organization and evolution of variable region genes of the human immunoglobulin heavy chain. J. molec. Biol. *190:* 529–541 (1986).

32 Berman, J.E.; Mellis, S.J.; Pollock, R.; et al.: Content and organization of the human Ig VH locus. Definition of three new VH families and linkage to the Ig CH locus. Eur. molec. Biol. Org. J. *7:* 727–738 (1988).

33 Lee, K.H.; Matsuda, F.; Kinashi, T.; Kodaira, M.; Honjo, T.: A novel family of variable region genes of the human immunoglobulin heavy chain. J. molec. Biol. *195:* 761–768 (1987).

34 Malynn, B.A.; Berman, J.E.; Yancopoulos, G.D.; Bona, C.A.; Alt, F.W.: Expression of the immunoglobulin heavy-chain variable gene repertoire. Curr. Top. Microbiol. Immunol. *135:* 75–94 (1987).

35 Shen, A.; Humphries, C.; Tucker, P.; Blattner, F.: Human heavy-chain variable region gene family nonrandomly rearranged in familial chronic lymphocytic leukemia. Proc. natn. Acad. Sci. USA *84:* 8563–8567 (1987).

36 Schroeder, H.W., Jr.; Hillson, J.L.; Perlmutter, R.M.: Early restriction of the human antibody repertoire. Science *238:* 791–793 (1987).

37 Milstein, C.: Linked groups of residues in immunoglobulin k chains. Nature, Lond. *216:* 330–332 (1967).

38 Wang, A.C.; Fudenberg, H.H.; Wells, J.V.: A new subgroup of the Kappa chain variable region associated with anti-Pr cold agglutinins. Nature New Biol. *243:* 126–128 (1973).

39 Hood, L.; Ein, D.: Immunoglobulin lambda chain structure: two genes, one polypeptide chain. Nature, Lond. *220:* 764–767 (1968).

40 Tischendorf, F.W.; Tischendorf, M.M.; Osserman, E.F.: Subgroup-specific antigenic

marker on immunoglobulin lambda chains: identification of three subtypes of the variable region. J. Immun. *105:* 1033–1035 (1970).

41 Solomon, A.: Light chains of immunoglobulins: structural-genetic correlates. Blood *68:* 603–610 (1986).

42 Poljak, R.J.: Three-dimensional structure, function and genetic control of immuno-globulins. Nature, Lond. *256:* 373–376 (1975).

43 Padlan, E.A.; Davies, D.R.: Variability of three-dimensional structure in immuno-globulins. Proc. natn. Acad. Sci. USA *72:* 819–823 (1975).

44 Segal, D.M.; Padlan, E.A.; Cohen, G.H.; Rudikoff, S.; Potter, M.; Davies, D.R.: The three-dimensional structure of a phosphorylcholine-binding mouse immunoglobulin Fab and the nature of the antigen binding site. Proc. natn. Acad. Sci. USA *71:* 4298–4302 (1974).

45 Poljak, R.J.: X-ray diffraction studies of immunoglobulins. Adv. Immunol. *21:* 1–33 (1975).

46 Alzari, P.M.; Lascombe, M.B.; Poljak, R.J.: Three-dimensional structure of anti-bodies. A. Rev. Immunol. *6:* 555–580 (1988).

47 Greenstein, J.L.; Solomon, A.; Abraham, G.N.: Monoclonal antibodies reactive with idiotypic and variable-region specific determinants on human immunoglobulins. Immunology *51:* 17–25 (1984).

48 Posnett, D.N.; Wisniewolski, R.; Pernis, B.; Kunkel, H.G.: Dissection of the human antigammaglobulin idiotype system with monoclonal antibodies. Scand. J. Im-munol *23:* 169–181 (1986).

49 Silverman, G.J.; Carson, D.A.; Solomon, A.; Fong, S.: Human kappa light chain subgroup analysis with synthetic peptide-induced antisera. J. immunol. Methods *95:* 249–257 (1986).

50 Silverman, G.J.; Goldfien, R.D.; Chen, P.; et al.: Idiotypic and subgroup analysis of human monoclonal rheumatoid factors. Implications for structural and genetic basis of autoantibodies in humans. J. clin. Invest. *82:* 469–475 (1988).

51 Miller, R.A.; Maloney, D.G.; Warnke, R.; Levy, R.: Treatment of B-cell lymphoma with monoclonal anti-idiotype antibody. New Engl. J. Med. *306:* 517–522 (1982).

52 Meeker, T.C.; Lowder, J.; Maloney, D.G.; et al.: A clinical trial of anti-idiotype therapy for B cell malignancy. Blood *65:* 1349–1363 (1985).

53 Lowder, J.N.; Meeker, T.C.; Campbell, M.; et al.: Studies on B lymphoid tumors treated with monoclonal anti-idiotype antibodies. Correlation with clinical re-sponses. Blood *69:* 199–210 (1987).

54 Dillman, R.O.; Shawler, D.L.; Sobol, R.E.; et al.: Murine monoclonal antibody therapy in two patients with chronic lymphocytic leukemia. Blood *59:* 1036–1045 (1982).

55 Levy, R.; Levy, S.; Cleary, M.L.; et al.: Somatic mutation in human B-cell tumors. Immunol. Rev. *96:* 43–58 (1987).

56 Meeker, T.; Lowder, J.; Cleary, M.L.; et al.: Emergence of idiotype variants during treatment of B-cell lymphoma with anti-idiotype antibodies. New Engl. J. Med. *312:* 1658–1665 (1985).

57 Sklar, J.; Cleary, M.L.; Thielemans, K.; Gralow, J.; Warnke, R.; Levy, R.: Biclonal B-cell lymphoma. New Engl. J. Med. *311:* 20–27 (1984).

58 Cleary, M.L.; Galili, N.; Trela, M.; Levy, R.; Sklar, J.: Single cell origin of bigeno-typic and biphenotypic B cell proliferations in human follicular lymphomas. J. exp. Med. *167:* 582–597 (1988).

59 Cleary, M.L.; Meeker, T.C.; Levy, S.; et al.: Clustering of extensive somatic muta-

tions in the variable region of an immunoglobulin heavy chain gene from a human B cell lymphoma. Cell *44:* 97–106 (1986).

60 Griffiths, G.M.; Berek, C.; Kaartinen, M.; Milstein, C.: Somatic mutation and the maturation of immune response to 2-phenyl oxazolone. Nature, Lond. *312:* 271–275 (1984).

61 Clarke, S.H.; Huppi, K.; Ruezinsky, D.; Staudt, L.; Gerhard, W.; Weigert, M.: Inter- and intraclonal diversity in the antibody response to influenza hemagglutinin. J. exp. Med. *161:* 687–704 (1985).

62 Raffeld, M.; Neckers, L.; Longon, D.L.; Cossman, J.: Spontaneous alteration of idiotype in a monoclonal B-cell lymphoma. Escape from detection by anti-idiotype. New Engl. J. Med. *312:* 1653–1658 (1985).

63 Carroll, W.L.; Lowder, J.N.; Streifer, R.; Warnke, R.; Levy, S.; Levy, R.: Idiotype variant cell populations in patients with B cell lymphoma. J. exp. Med. *164:* 1566–1580 (1986).

64 Kunkel, H.G.; Agnello, V.; Winchester, R.J.; Capra, J.D.; Kehoe, J.M.: Cross-idiotypic specificity among monoclonal IgM proteins with anti-globulin activity. Proc. natn. Acad. Sci. USA *71:* 4032–4036 (1974).

65 Carson, D.A.; Fong, S.: A common idiotope on human rheumatoid factors identified by a hybridoma antibody. Molec. Immunol. *20:* 1081–1087 (1983).

66 Mageed, R.A.; Dearlove, M.; Goodall, D.M.; Jefferis, R.: Immunogenic and antigenic epitopes of immunoglobulins XVII – Monoclonal antibodies reactive with common and restricted idiotopes to the heavy chain of human rheumatoid factors. Rheumatol. int. *6:* 179–183 (1986).

67 Kunkel, H.G.; Winchester, R.J.; Joslin, F.G.; Capra, J.D.: Similarities in the light chains of anti-gamma-globulins showing cross-idiotypic specificities. J. exp. Med. *139:* 128–136 (1974).

68 Andrews, D.W.; Capra, J.D.: Complete amino acid sequence of variable domains from two monoclonal human anti-gamma globulins of the Wa cross-idiotypic group: suggestion that the J segments are involved in the structural correlate of the idiotype. Proc. natn. Acad. Sci. USA *78:* 3799–3803 (1981).

69 Ledford, D.K.; Goni, F.; Pizzolato, M.; Franklin, E.C.; Solomon, A.; Frangione, B.: Preferential association of kappa IIIb light chains with monoclonal human IgM kappa autoantibodies. J. Immun. *131:* 1322–1325 (1983).

70 Capra, J.D.; Kehoe, J.M.: Structure of antibodies with shared idiotypy: the complete sequence of the heavy chain variable regions of two immunoglobulin M anti-gamma globulins. Proc. natn. Acad. Sci. USA *71:* 4032–4036 (1974).

71 Pons-Estel, :B.; Goni, F.; Solomon, A.; Frangione, B.: Sequence similarities among kappa IIIb chains of monoclonal human IgM kappa autoantibodies. J. exp. Med. *160:* 893–904 (1984).

72 Capra, J.D.; Kehoe, J.M.; Williams, R.C., Jr.; Feizi, T.; Kunkel, H.G.: Light chain sequences of human IgM cold agglutinins (variable-region subgroups amino-acid sequence-kappa light chain-N-terminal). Proc. natn. Acad. Sci. USA *69:* 40–43 (1972).

73 Kipps, T.J.; Fong, S.; Tomhave, E.; Chen, P.P.; Goldfien, R.D.; Carson, D.A.: High-frequency expression of a conserved kappa light-chain variable-region gene in chronic lymphocytic leukemia. Proc. natn. Acad. Sci. USA *84:* 2916–2920 (1987).

74 Kipps, T.J.; Fong, S.; Tomhave, E.; Chen, P.P.; Goldfien, R.D.; Carson, D.A.: Immunoglobulin V gene utilization in CLL; in Gale, Rai, Chronic lymphocytic leukemia: recent progress and future direction, pp. 115–126 (Liss, New York 1987).

75 Carson, D.A.; Chen, P.P.; Kipps, T.J.; et al.: Molecular basis for the cross-reactive

idiotypes on human anti-IgG autoantibodies (rheumatoid factors). Ciba Fdn Symp. *129:* 123–134 (197).

76 Carson, D.A.; Chen, P.P.; Kipps, T.J.; et al.: Idiotypic and genetic studies of human rheumatoid factors. Arthritis Rheum. *30:* 1321–1325 (1987).

77 Kipps, T.J.; Robins, B.A.; Kuster, P.; Carson, D.A.: Autoantibody-associated cross-reactive idiotypes expressed at high frequency in chronic lymphocytic leukemia relative to B-cell lymphomas of follicular center cell origin. Blood *72:* 422–428 (1988).

78 Kipps, T.J.; Tomhave, E.; Chen, P.P.; Carson, D.A.: Autoantibody-associated kappa light chain variable region gene expressed in chronic lymphocytic leukemia with little or no somatic mutation. Implications for etiology and immunotherapy. J. exp. Med. *167:* 840–852 (1988).

79 Radoux, V.; Chen, P.P.; Sorge, J.A.; Carson, D.A.: A conserved human germline V kappa gene directly encodes rheumatoid factor light chains. J. exp. Med. *164:* 2119–2124 (1986).

80 Chen, P.P.; Albrandt, K.; Kipps, T.J.; Radoux, V.; Liu, F.T.; Carson, D.A.: Isolation and characterization of human VkIII germ-line genes. Implications for the molecular basis of human VkIII light chain diversity. J. Immun. *139:* 1727–1733 (1987).

81 Chen, P.P.; Robbins, D.L.; Jirik, F.R.; Kipps, T.J.; Carson, D.A.: Isolation and characterization of a light chain variable region gene for human rheumatoid factors. J. exp. Med. *166:* 1900–1905 (1987).

82 Kipps, T.J.; Tomhave, E.; Pratt, L.F.; Chen, P.P.; Carson, D.A.: Developmentally restricted VH gene expressed at high frequency in chronic lymphocytic leukemia. Proc. natn. Acad. Sci. USA (in press, 1989).

83 Newkirk, M.M.; Mageed, R.A.; Jefferis, R.; Chen, P.P.; Capra, J.D.: Complete amino acid sequences of variable regions of two human IgM rheumatoid factors, BOR and KAS of the Wa idiotypic family, reveal restricted use of heavy and light chain variable and joining region gene segments. J. exp. Med. *166:* 550–564 (1987).

84 Preud'homme, J.L.; Seligmann, M.: Anti-human immunoglobulin G activity of membrane-bound immunoglobulin M in lymphoproliferative disorders. Proc. natn. Acad. Sci. USA *69:* 2132–2125 (1972).

85 Mann, D.L.; DeSantis, P.; Mark, G.; et al.: HTLV-I-associated B-cell CLL: indirect role for retrovirus in leukemogenesis. Science *236:* 1103–1106 (1987).

86 Newkirk, M.M.; Gram, H.; Heinrich, G.F.; Ostberg, L.; Capra, J.D.; Wasserman, R.L.: Complete protein sequences of the variable regions of the cloned heavy and light chains of a human anti-cytomegalovirus antibody reveal a striking similarity to human monoclonal rheumatoid factors of the Wa idiotypic family. J. clin. Invest. *81:* 1511–1518 (1988).

87 Boumsell, L.; Coppin, H.; Pham, D.; et al.: An antigen shared by a human T cell subset and B cell chronic lymphocytic leukemic cells. Distribution on normal and malignant lymphoid cells. J. exp. Med. *152:* 229–234 (1980).

88 Wang, C.Y.; Good, R.A.; Ammirati, P.; Dymbort, G.; Evans, R.L.: Identification of a p69,71 complex expressed on human T cells sharing determinants with B-type chronic lymphatic leukemic cells. J. exp. Med. *151:* 1539–1544 (1980).

89 Martin, P.J.; Hansen, J.A.; Nowinski, R.C.; Brown, M.A.: A new human T-cell differentiation antigen. Unexpected expression on chronic lymphocytic leukemia cells. Immunogenetics *11:* 429–439 (1980).

90 Royston, I.; Majda, J.A.; Baird, S.M.; Meserve, B.L.; Griffiths, J.C.: Human T cell antigens defined by monoclonal antibodies: the 65,000-dalton antigen of T cells

(T65) is also found on chronic lymphocytic leukemia cells bearing surface immuno-globulin. J. Immun. *125:* 725–731 (1980).

91 Martin, P.J.; Hansen, J.A.; Siadak, A.W.; Nowinski, R.C.: Monoclonal antibodies recognizing normal human T lymphocytes and malignant human B lymphocytes: a comparative study. J. Immun. *127:* 1920–1923 (1981).

92 Gobbi, M.; Caligaris-Cappio, F.; Janossy, G.: Normal equivalent cells of B cell malignancies: analysis with monoclonal antibodies. Br. J. Haematol. *54:* 393–403 (1983).

93 Caligaris-Cappio, F.; Gobbi, M.; Gofill, M.; Janossy, G.: Infrequent normal B lymphocytes express features of B-chronic lymphocytic leukemia. J. exp. Med. *155:* 623–628 (1982).

94 Gadol, N.; Ault, K.A.: Phenotypic and functional characterization of human Leu1 (CD5) cells. Immunol. Rev. *93:* 23–34 (1986).

95 Hardy, R.R.; Hayakawa, K.: Development and physiology of Ly-1 B and its human homolog, B. Immunol. Rev. *93:* 53–79 (1986).

96 Kipps, T.J.; Vaughan, J.H.: Genetic influence on the levels of circulating CD5 B lymphocytes. J. Immun. *139:* 1060–1064 (1987).

97 Hayakawa, K.; Hardy, R.R.; Honda, M.; Herzenberg, L.A.; Steinberg, A.D.: Ly-1 B cells: functionally distinct lymphocytes that secrete IgM autoantibodies. Proc. natn. Acad. Sci. USA *81:* 2494–2498 (1984).

98 Herzenberg, L.A.; Stall, A.M.; Lalor, P.A.; Sidman, C.; Moore, W.A.; Parks, D.R.: The Ly-1 B cell lineage. Immunol. Rev. *93:* 81–102 (1986).

99 Hayakawa, K.; Hardy, R.R.; Parks, D.R.; Herzenberg, L.A.: The 'Ly-1' B cell subpopulation in normal immunodefective, and autoimmune mice. J. exp. Med. *157:* 202–218 (1983).

100 Okumura, K.; Hayakawa, K.; Tada, T.: Cell-to-cell interaction controlled by im-munoglobulin genes of Thy-1−, Lyt-1+, Ig+ (B′) cell in allotype-restricted antibody production. J. exp. Med. *156:* 443–453 (1982).

101 Sherr, D.H.; Dorf, M.E.: An idiotype-specific helper population that bears immuno-globulin, Ia, and Lyt-1 determinants. J. exp. Med. *159:* 1189–1200 (1984).

102 Sherr, D.H.; Dorf, M.E.; Gibson, M.; Sidman, C.L.: Ly-1 B helper cells in autoim-mune 'viable motheaten' mice. J. Immun. *139:* 1811–1817 (1987).

103 Sherr, D.H.; Braun, J.; Dorf, M.E.: Idiotype-specific Ly-1 B cell-mediated helper activity: hybridomas that produce anti-idiotype antibody and nonimmunoglobulin lymphokine(s)1. J. Immun. *138:* 2057–2062 (1987).

104 Paglieroni, T.; Caggiano, V.; MacKenzie, M.: CD5 positive immunoregulatory B cell subsets. Am. J. Hematol. *28:* 276–278 (1988).

105 MacKenzie, M.R.; Paglieroni, T.G.; Warner, N.L.: Multiple myeloma: an immuno-logic profile. IV. The EA rosette-forming cell is a Leu-1 positive immunoregulatory B cell. J. Immun. *139:* 24–28 (1987).

106 Casali, P.; Burastero, S.E.; Nakamura, M.; Inghirami, G.; Notkins, A.L.: Human lymphocytes making rheumatoid factor and antibody to belong to Leu-1+ B-cell subset. Science *236:* 77–81 (1987).

107 Hardy, R.R.; Hayakawa, K.; Shimizu, M.; Yamasaki, K.; Kishimoto, T.: Rheuma-toid factor secretion from human Leu-1+ B cells. Science *236:* 81–83 (1987).

108 Bofill, M.; Janossy, G.; Janossa, M.; et al.: Human B cell development. II. Subpopu-lations in the human. J. Immun. *134:* 1531–1538 (1985).

109 Antin, J.H.; Emerson, S.G.; Martin, P.; Gadol, N.; Ault, K.A.: Leu-1+ (CD5+) B cells.

A major lymphoid subpopulation in fetal spleen: phenotypic and functional studies. J. Immun. *136:* 505–510 (1986).

110 Kipps, T.J.; Rassenti, L.A.; Pratt, L.F.; Chen, P.P.; Carson, D.A.: Frequent immuno-globulin gene rearrangement of a conserved kappa light chain variable region gene in chronic lymphocytic leukemia (Abstract). Blood *72s:* 208a (1988).

111 Alt, F.W.; Yancopoulos, G.D.; Blackwell, T.K.; et al.: Ordered rearrangement of immunoglobulin heavy chain variable region segments. Eur. molec. Biol. Org. J. *3:* 1209–1219 (1984).

112 Yancopoulos, G.D.; Alt, F.W.: Developmentally controlled and tissue-specific ex-pression of unrearranged VH gene segments. Cell *40:* 271–281 (1985).

113 Alt, F.W.; Blackwell, T.K.; Yancopoulos, G.D.: Development of the primary anti-body repertoire. Science *238:* 1079–1087 (1987).

114 Pohlenz, H.D.; Straubinger, B.; Thiebe, R.; Pech, M.; Zimmer, F.J.; Zachau, H.G.: The human V kappa locus. Characterization of extended immunoglobulin gene regions by cosmid cloning. J. molec. Biol. *193:* 241–253 (1987).

115 Humphries, C.G.; Shen, A.; Kuziel, W.A.; Capra, J.D.; Blattner, F.R.; Tucker, P.W.: A new human immunoglobulin VH family preferentially rearranged in immature B-cell tumours. Nature, Lond. *331:* 446–449 (1988).

116 Stevenson, F.K.; Wrightham, M.; Glennie, M.J.; et al.: Antibodies to shared idiotypes as agents for analysis and therapy for human B cell tumors. Blood *68:* 430–436 (1986).

117 Burns, B.F.; Warnke, R.A.; Doggett, R.S.; Rouse, R.V.: Expression of a T-cell antigen (Leu-1) by B-cell lymphomas. Am. J. Path. *113:* 165–171 (1983).

118 Knowles, D.M., II; Halper, J.P.; Azzo, W.; Wang, C.Y.: Reactivity of monoclonal antibodies Leu 1 and OKT1 with malignant human lymphoid cells. Correlation with conventional cell markers. Cancer *52:* 1369–1377 (1983).

119 Cossman, J.; Neckers, L.M.; Hsu, S.; Longo, D.; Jaffe, E.S.: Low-grade lymphomas. Expression of developmentally regulated B-cell antigens. Am. J. Path. *115:* 117–124 (1984).

120 Al Saati, T.; Laurent, G.; Caveriviere, P.; Rigal, F.; Delsol, G.: Reactivity of Leu 1 and T101 monoclonal antibodies with B cell lymphomas (correlations with other immunological markers). Clin. exp. Immunol. *58:* 631–638 (1984).

121 Medeiros, L.J.; Strickler, J.G.; Picker, L.J.; Gelb, A.B.; Weiss, L.M.; Warnke, R.A.: 'Well-differentiated' lymphocytic neoplasms. Immunologic findings correlated with clinical presentation and morphologic features. Am. J. Path. *129:* 523–535 (1987).

122 Oord, J.J. van den; Wolf-Peeters, C., de; Pulford, K.A.; Mason, D.Y.; Desmet, V.J.: Mantle zone lymphoma. Immuno- and enzymehistochemical studies on the cell of origin. Am. J. surg. Pathol. *10:* 780–788 (1986).

123 Kipps, T.J.; Robbins, B.A.; Meisenholder, G.W.; Carson, D.A.; Banks, P.: Autoanti-body-associated cross reactive idiotypes expressed at high frequencies in CD5-positive non-Hodgkin's B cell lymphomas (Abstract). Blood *72s:* 245a (1988).

124 Giardina, S.L.; Schroff, R.W.; Kipps, T.J.; et al.: The generation of monoclonal anti-idiotype antibodies to human B cell-derived leukemias and lymphomas. J. Immun. *135:* 653–658 (1985).

Thomas J. Kipps, MD, PhD, Department of Molecular and Experimental Medicine, Scripps Clinic and Research Foundation, 10666 North Torrey Pines Road, La Jolla, CA 92037 (USA)

Carson DA, Chen PP, Kipps TJ (eds): Idiotypes in Biology and Medicine.
Chem Immunol. Basel, Karger, 1990, vol 48, pp 185–208

Structure and Regulation of Internal Image Idiotypes

William V. Williams[a], *H. Robert Guy*[b], *Jeffrey A. Cohen*[c],
David B. Weiner[a], *Mark I. Greene*[a]

[a]Department of Pathology and Laboratory Medicine and
[c]Department of Neurology, University of Pennsylvania School of Medicine,
Philadelphia, Pa., USA; [b]Laboratory of Mathematical Biology,
National Cancer Institutes of Health, Bethesda, Md., USA

Introduction

Antibody molecules have the ability to bind a wide range of chemically dissimilar antigens. While the most common antigens are proteins, antibodies can also bind carbohydrates, biopolymers, small chemicals (haptens), and certain lipids. Protein antigens themselves are also extremely diverse in both primary, secondary, and tertiary structure. The antigenic sites of certain proteins have been extensively characterized [1]. These studies indicate that virtually any site on the surface of a protein that is accessible to an antibody-variable region can be antigenic [1]. The extent of variation inherent in protein structure is extensive (i.e. 20 different amino acids aligned in any order and able to fold into multiple conformations in a three-dimensional space). It is clear that antibody molecules must exhibit similar structural diversity.

Antibodies are able to achieve this structural heterogeneity by utilizing specific regions in a three-dimensional space. The general structure of a typical dimeric antibody molecule is depicted in figure 1. Two heavy and two light chains combine to form a tetramer bound by disulfide bridges. The heavy and light chains are composed of distinct constant and variable regions. Three-dimensional analysis of antibody molecules [2–4] reveals that the variable region and distinct subunits of the constant region share a

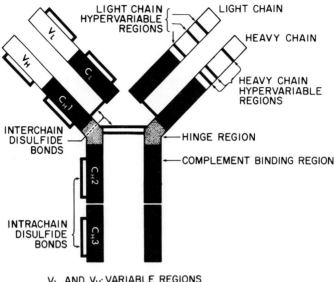

VL AND VH: VARIABLE REGIONS
CL AND CH: CONSTANT REGIONS

Fig. 1. General structure of an immunoglobulin molecule. The constant and variable regions with the heavy and light chains are indicated. The positions of the hypervariable regions within the variable regions is shown. Modified from Wasserman and Capa (with permission) [78].

pleated sheets (fig. 2). The heavy and light chain variable regions each have this general structure, as do the heavy and light chain constant regions.

The structure of a particular antibody antigen-combining region is included within the idiotypic portion of that antibody. The idiotypic portion of an antibody molecule typically resides within the variable region. This includes several hypervariable loops which project outward from the antiparallel beta-pleated sheet structure (fig. 2, 3). Three hypervariable loops are contributed by the heavy and three by the light chain variable regions. It is within these loops that the structural diversity of antibody molecules is manifested.

The diversity of antibody molecules can be utilized to probe a number of biologic systems. Antibodies can be developed which functionally mimic other molecules. The network theory of Jerne [5] predicted that an antibody could develop which binds to the idiotype/antigen-combining site of another antibody molecule. This sort of antibody, which is termed an anti-

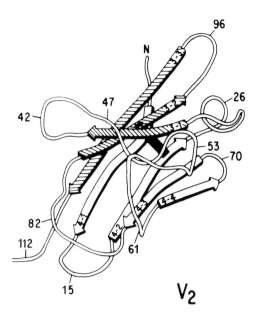

Fig. 2. Schematic with an immunoglobulin light chain variable region domain. The conserved region consists of the anti-parallel beta-pleated sheets. Hypervariable loops are represented by residues 26 (CDR I), 53 (CDR II), and 96 (CDR III). Modified from Edmundson et al. (with permission) [3].

idiotypic antibody or anti-idiotype, is predicted to have certain properties. In particular, an antigen bound by a particular antigen-combining region (idiotype) may be functionally mimicked by an anti-idiotypic antibody that also binds to the same region of that idiotype. Anti-idiotypic antibodies that mimic antigens in this way are said to bear the 'internal image' of the antigen.

This internal image mimickry has been utilized in a number of systems to analyze receptor-ligand interactions [6]. Internal image anti-idiotypes have been developed against a number of ligands, and these anti-idiotypes mimic the ligands by specifically combining with their receptors. Anti-idiotypic/antireceptor antibodies have been developed which recognize specific receptors for retinol-binding protein [7, 8], insulin [9, 10], beta-adrenergic catecholamines [11, 12], the formyl chemotactic peptide Fmet-leu-phe [13], beta-1-H globulin [14], thyroid-stimulating hormone [15], and the mammalian reovirus type 3 [16–19]. These anti-idiotypic/antireceptor antibodies can mimic ligands both structurally and functionally.

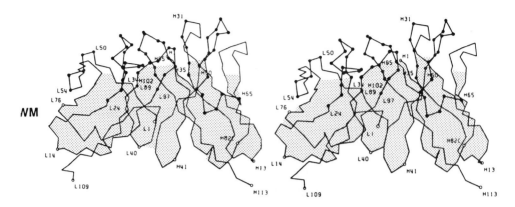

Fig. 3. Stereoview of the amino acid backbone of the variable region of the immunoglobulin NEWM. The conserved portion is shaded in, while portions of the hypervariable loops are unshaded. Modified from Kabat et al. (with permission) [79].

Since anti-idiotypic antibodies can arise during a primary immune response [20], it follows that during the development of an immune response to a pathogen, anti-idiotypic antibodies may arise which bind to the receptor for that pathogen. These anti-idiotypes would bear the internal image of the receptor-interaction site of the pathogen. The development of receptor-binding anti-idiotypic antibodies (which would be autoantibodies) might be deleterious to the host. It is likely that the expression of internal image antibodies of this type would be regulated.

Prior studies have described anti-idiotypic antireceptor antibodies which bear the internal image of the receptor interaction site of reovirus type 3. These studies have led to insights into the structural basis for internal image mimickry as well as into regulation of antibody development.

The Reovirus System

The mammalian reoviruses are ubiquitous enteric cytopathogenic viruses which are members of the picornaviridae [21]. Reoviruses consist of three serologically distinguishable subgroups: strain 1 (prototype Lang), strain 2 (prototype Jones), and strain 3 (prototype Dearing). Reovirus particles possess a double capsid structure, each capsid arranged in distinct morphological subunits or capsomeres [22]. The viral genome is contained within the inner capsid which is highly resistant to protease digestion. The outer capside is relatively labile to proteases and this differential sensitivity influences the processing of the reovirus to the infective state [23]. The reovirus genome consists of ten dsRNA segments which exist in three size classes designated large (L), medium (M), and small (S). Each genomic segment transcribes a unique mRNA, designated l, m, and s, which is in turn translated into the peptides designated lambda, mu and sigma. The outer capsid is composed of the polypeptides mu 1c, sigma 3, sigma 1, and the spike-associated protein lambda 2. These proteins play a major role in defining the patterns of viral tropism and pathogenesis. Due to the segmented nature of the reovirus genome, viral recombinants are readily generated upon mixed infection [24]. Intertypic recombinants have been used to correlate the genome segments between serotypes 1, 2 and 3, to identify the genomic segments that encode various viral polypeptides, and to define viral segments relevant to pathogenesis [24–26].

Reovirus Pathogenesis and Tropism

Despite overall structural similarity, the three serotypes of reovirus mediate different diseases. Type 3 reovirus is most probably spread through peripheral or olfactory neurons to the central nervous system [27]. Type 1 virus appears to be spread by the blood and lymphatics [28]. Type 1 infection results in the infection of the ependymal cells which line the ventricular cavities and has no effect on neurons [29]. In contrast, inoculation of neonatal mice with reovirus 3 results in acute destruction of neurons of the pyramidal regions of the hippocampus and other areas of the brain, resulting in fatal encephalitis [30, 31].

Tropism has been shown to map to the S1 gene segment which encodes the virion outer capsid protein sigma 1 which also serves as the hemagglutinin (HA) [24–26]. Recombinants which contain the genome of type 1 with the exception of the hemagglutinin of type 3, designated 1HA3, display the tropism of type 3 virus. The reciprocal recombinant, 3HA1, mimics type 1 tropism. Binding of intact virus has been shown to occur through the interaction of the hemagglutinin with specific high-affinity cell surface receptors [16, 32, 33].

Binding studies utilizing radiolabelled reovirus particles have indicated that reovirus types 1 and 3 utilize distinct receptors on most cells [18]. Mouse fibroblasts (L cells) which bear receptors for both reovirus types 1 and 3 have distinct receptors for each serotype [33]. Certain murine T cell lines bear receptors for reovirus type 3 but not reovirus type 1 [18]. In contrast, intestinal epithelial cells bear receptors for reovirus type 1 but not reovirus type 3 [34]. Use of reassortant reovirus particles has allowed these interactions to be mapped to the S1 gene segment.

Infection with reovirus type 3 also affects host cell macromolecular synthesis. In L cells a dramatic inhibition of DNA synthesis occurs 8 h after infection [35]. UV-inactivated reovirus 3 can also inhibit DNA synthesis indicating that the process does not depend on viral replication [36]. Recent studies have indicated that this effect is due to receptor perturbation and aggregation [67].

Mapping of the Reovirus Type 3 HA

The topologic structure of the reovirus type 3 HA (HA3) has been studied by utilizing a panel of monoclonal antibodies that bind the HA3. It was possible to delineate distinct domains within the HA3 responsible for hemagglutination and viral neutralization [37]. While some antibodies were found that affected both neutralization and hemagglutination, several were noted to affect these processes independently. Competitive binding studies indicated that these domains are physically distinct, but located close to one another on the HA3 subunit [38].

One neutralizing monoclonal antibody (9BG5) was of particular interest. The 9BG5 antibody, developed in Balb/c mice, was found to strongly bind the HA3, and to neutralize reovirus type 3 infectivity without affecting reovirus type 1 [37, 38]. Treatment of reovirus type 3 particles with 9BG5 rendered them incapable of attaching to cells [39]. These observations implied that 9BG5 bound the HA3 at or near the site that attaches to the cellular receptor for reovirus type 3.

Initial Development of Anti-Idiotypes to Reovirus Type 3

In order to better characterize the interactions between reovirus type 3 and its receptor, anti-idiotypic antibodies were developed to mimic the HA3. Initially, these anti-idiotypes were developed by immunizing rabbits with polyclonal antireovirus type 3 antibodies developed in infected mice [16, 40]. These were initially screened for their ability to inhibit the binding of anti-HA3 antibodies to the HA3. These rabbit anti-idiotypes (termed anti-ID3) displayed a dominant idiotypic reactivity, represented by the 9BG5 idiotype.

In a series of studies, it was established that anti-ID3 specifically recognized a cell-surface structure that acted as the receptor for reovirus type 3 [16, 17, 40]. Thus, anti-ID3 was able to stain cells bearing reovirus type 3 receptors on flow cytometry [40], and competed with HA3 for binding to these cells [6].

These studies indicated that anti-ID3, which mimicked the HA3, was strongly recognized by the monoclonal neutralizing antibody 9BG5. This implied that an anti-idiotype developed against 9BG5 might behave similarly. This approach was taken for the development of monoclonal internal image idiotypes of reovirus type 3.

Development of Monoclonal Anti-Idiotype to Reovirus Type 3

To minimize allotypic reactivities which might arise, anti-idiotypes to 9BG5 were developed in syngeneic Balb/c mice. Hybridomas were generated from 9BG5 immune Balb/c mice and screened for their ability to bind 9BG5 [18]. One hybridoma, termed 87.92.6, was found to bind 9BG5 and to inhibit the interactions between 9BG5 and the HA3. Absorption of 87.92.6 with reovirus type 3 receptor-bearing cells eliminated its binding to 9BG5 [18]. It was felt that 87.92.6 was likely to be the 'internal image' of the receptor interaction site of the HA3.

Staining of a panel of cells with 87.92.6 revealed that its binding pattern mirrored that of reovirus type 3 [18]. In addition, prior incubation of cells with 87.92.6 inhibited the binding of reovirus type 3 particles [18, 41]. This indicated that 87.92.6 specifically interacted with the reovirus type 3 receptor on these cells. It was felt that 87.92.6 was likely to bear within its variable region structure an internal image of the HA3 receptor interaction site.

Characterization of the Reovirus Type 3 Receptor

By utilizing anti-ID3 it was possible to biochemically characterize the reovirus type 3 receptor on several cells [17, 41]. Immunoprecipitation studies revealed a 65,000-dalton glycoprotein with a pI of 5.9. This structure was found to possess N-linked glycosylation sites. Electrophoretic immunoblot studies revealed that this was the only cell-surface structure recognized by both reovirus type 3 and the antireceptor antibodies [17, 41]. Comparison of the reovirus receptor on murine thymoma (R1.1) and rat neuroblastoma

(B104) cells indicated that similar structures on the cell surface are recognized by the reovirus type 3 and the antireceptor antibodies, as suggested from cellular and binding studies. This receptor was found on mouse, rat, monkey and human cells. Furthermore, diverse tissue types, including lymphoid and neuronal cells, express the receptor structure.

Structural Similarity of the Reovirus Type 3 and Beta-2-Adrenergic Receptors

The reovirus type 3 receptor is structurally similar to the mammalian beta-adrenergic receptor [42, 43]. This conclusion is based on the following observations: (i) purified beta-adrenergic receptor is immunoprecipitable by antireovirus type 3 receptor antibody [42]; (ii) purified reovirus type 3 receptor obtained from murine thymoma cells and beta-adrenergic receptor obtained from calf lung exhibit identical molecular masses and isoelectric points [42]; (iii) tryptic digests of purified reovirus type 3 and beta-adrenergic receptors display indistinguishable fragment patterns [42]; (iv) purified reovirus type 3 receptor binds the beta-adrenergic selective antagonist [^{125}I]-iodohydroxybenzylpindolol and this binding is blocked by the beta-agonist isoproterenol [42, 43].

The mammalian beta-2-adrenergic protein is encoded by a member of a gene family that encodes receptors that have multiple membrane-spanning units. This family includes the reovirus type 3 receptor [42, 43], beta-2- [44, 45] and beta-1- [46] adrenergic receptors, muscarinic acetylcholine receptor [47], rhodopsin [48, 49], bacteriorhodopsin [50], opsin blue [51], opsin green [51], the alpha and beta mating factor receptors of the yeast *Saccharomyces cerevisiaee* [52, 53], the mas oncogene [54], and the enzyme HMG-CoA reductase [55]. These proteins share many structural similarities, but the overall organization into multiple membrane spanning regions is by far the most characteristic.

Immunologic Mimicking of the HA3 by 87.92.6

The above studies indicated a likely structural similarity between 87.92.6 and the HA3 in their interactions with the reovirus type 3 receptor. This structural similarity is also manifest in their interactions with the immune system. In several studies performed in syngeneic Balb/c mice it was demonstrated that both T cells and B cells specific for reovirus type 3 specifically recognized 87.92.6 [56–58]. Mice primed with 87.92.6 developed delayed-type hypersensitivity T cells (T_{DTH}) specific for reovirus type 3, but not reovirus type 1 [56]. Cytotoxic T lymphocytes (CTL) specific for reovirus type 3 were able to lyse 87.92.6-bearing hybridoma cells [57]. These two observations are of interest in that CTL and T_{DTH} are likely to be recognizing processed fragments of reovirus type 3 or 87.92.6 in association with major histocompatibility molecules. This would imply that these processed fragments must also bear similar structures. In addition, processed fragments of 87.92.6 are likely to be present on the surface of 87.92.6 hybridoma cells.

Syngeneic Balb/c mice primed with 87.92.6 develop antibodies that bind reovirus type 3 [58]. These antibodies had serotype-specific neutralizing activity against reovirus type 3 without affecting reovirus type 1. This confirmed that the site of the HA3 mimicked by 87.92.6 was a neutralizing epitope. It further implied close structural similarity between these two molecules as perceived by antibodies.

Amino Acid Sequence Similarity between the HA3 and 87.92.6

To probe the molecular basis for the structural similarity between 87.92.6 and the HA3, sequences of both the heavy chain and light chain variable regions (V_H and V_L respectively) of 87.92.6 were determined [59]. This study utilized primer extension sequencing of cDNA and deduction of the amino acid sequence. When these sequences were compared with the HA3 sequence [60], it was found that amino acids 317–332 of the HA3 shared sequence similarity with a combined determinant comprised of the 87.92.6 V_H and V_L second complementarity-determining regions (CDR II). As noted in table 1, the V_H CDRII shares sequence similarity with amino acids 317–325 of the HA3, while the V_L CDR II shares sequence similarity with amino acids 323–332 of the HA3.

A particularly high degree of sequence similarity was noted in the sequence Try-Ser-Gly-Ser, present in both the HA3 and the V_L CDR II. Application of the Chou and Fasman [61] algorithm to both the 87.92.6 and HA3 sequences indicated that this region is predicted to fold into a reverse turn, in both the HA3, and the 87.92.6 light chain CDR II. These observations focused attention on this region as the likely molecular correlate of the functional mimicking of the HA3 exhibited by 87.92.6. Synthetic peptides

Table 1. Amino acid sequence similarity between 87.92.6 and the reovirus HA3

V_H 43	Gln	Gly	Leu	Glu	Trp	Ilu	Gly	Arg	Ilu	Asp	Pro	Ala	Asn	Gly	56
	●	○	○		●	●	●		○						
Reo 317	Gln	Ser	Met	---	Trp	Ilu	Gly	Ilu	Val	Ser	Tyr	Ser	Gly	Ser	Gly	Leu	Asn	332
						○	○			●	●	●	●		●	○	
V_L 39	Lys	Pro	Gly	Lys	Thr	Asn	Lys	Leu	Leu	Ilu	Tyr	Ser	Gly	Ser	Thr	Leu	Gln	55

were utilized in a series of studies to further explore the significance of the sequence similarity.

9BG5 Binding to Synthetic Peptides

Four synthetic peptides were constructed to study the significance of this region. These are termed V_L peptide, V_H peptide, reo peptide, and V_H-V_L peptide. V_L peptide is composed of the amino acid sequence of the light chain CDR II of 87.92.6, V_H peptide corresponds to the heavy chain CDR II of 87.92.6, and reo peptide corresponds to amino acids 317–332 of the HA3 (table 1). V_H-V_L peptide was made by adding amino-terminal cysteine residues to both V_H and V_L peptides, and by covalently coupling them together [62].

Since monoclonal antibody 9BG5 binds to both the HA3 and 87.92.6, the ability of 9BG5 to bind these synthetic peptides was tested. In solid-phase radioimmunoassay (RIA), specific binding of 9BG5 to reo peptide, V_L peptide, and V_H-V_L peptide was demonstrated [62–65]. In this assay there was no significant binding to V_H peptide. However, V_H peptide was able to interact with 9BG5 in the liquid phase, as it could specifically inhibit binding of 9BG5 (fig. 4).

To establish the specificity of 9BG5 binding to these peptides, competitive binding studies were carried out (fig. 4). These indicated that binding of 9BG5 to reo peptide, V_L peptide and V_H-V_L peptide was specifically inhibited by preincubation of 9BG5 with V_L peptide or V_H peptide. A control peptide had no effect, and reo peptide was too poorly soluble for use in these assays. V_H-V_L peptide was consistently the most effective inhibitor in these assays. These results indicated that the binding of 9BG5 to these peptides was specific.

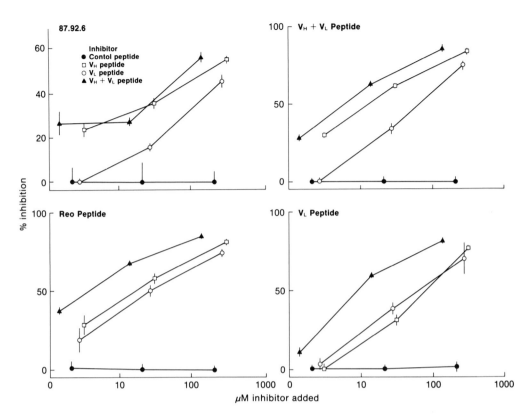

Fig. 4. Inhibition of 9BG5 binding by peptides. RIA plates were prepared as described [62]. Radioiodinated 9BG5 was incubated with the peptides and added to RIA wells for 30 min to 1 h. The wells were washed and counts per minute (cpm) bound was determined [62]. Percent inhibition of binding was calculated as described [62].

Peptide Inhibition of 9BG5 Binding to 87.92.6 and the HA3

Similar competition experiments were performed to study the specificity of the interactions between 9BG5 and both 87.92.6 and the HA3. Some of these data are shown in figure 4. In a competitive RIA where micotiter wells were coated with 87.92.6, increasing amounts of peptides were added to radiolabelled 9BG5, and the mixture added to the wells. V_L peptide and V_H peptide were able to inhibit 9BG5 binding. V_H-V_L peptide was again the most effective inhibitor of this interaction. This indicates that both the V_H CDR II and the V_L CDR II are likely to be involved in the interaction between 9BG5 and 87.92.6.

In a similar analysis, the ability of these peptides to inhibit the interaction of 9BG5 with the HA3 was measured. A slightly different result was obtained. V_L peptide markedly inhibited binding of radiolabelled reovirus type 3 to 9BG5. Several control peptides had no effect. V_H-V_L peptide was also effective, but no more effective than V_L peptide on a molar basis. V_H peptide did not effectively inhibit this interaction [62–65]. These results indicated that for the high-affinity binding of the HA3 to 9BG5, amino acids 323–332 of the HA3 are most important. These amino acids have the closest sequence similarity with V_L peptide. This epitope is likely to represent the neutralizing epitope recognized by 9BG5.

Peptide Inhibition of 87.92.6 and HA3 Binding to the Reovirus
Type 3 Receptor

In a similar series of experiments, the ability of the peptides to inhibit the binding of 87.92.6 and the HA3 to the reovirus type 3 receptor (Reo3R) was measured [62–65]. These results indicated that the interaction between these two ligands and the Reo3R was similar to the interaction between these ligands and 9BG5. Specifically, while V_L peptide contained the site most relevant to 87.92.6 binding to the Reo3R, V_H-V_L peptide was a more effective inhibitor of the interaction. However, V_L peptide was the most efficient inhibitor of HA3 binding to the Reo3R [62]. V_H peptide alone did not inhibit either of these interactions.

These results indicate that the same structural features involved in the interactions between 9BG5 and 87.92.6 are important in the Reo3R interaction with 87.92.6. Similarly, the interactions between 9BG5 and the HA3 have similar structural constraints as the interaction between the Reo3R and the HA3. Within these interactions, it was apparent that 9BG5 acted similarly to the Reo3R. 87.92.6 was also quite similar in its behavior to the HA3, as V_L peptide appeared to include the site most relevant to all these interactions. These inhibition studies are summarized in table 2.

From these studies it was concluded that V_L peptide likely contained the site most relevant to HA3 and 87.92.6 binding to both the Reo3R and 9BG5. The V_H peptide sequence seemed likely to play a role in correctly orienting the V_L peptide sequence for some of the interactions, while in others it played less of a role. Thus, the area of sequence similarity between the 87.92.6 V_L

Table 2. Summary of peptide inhibition studies[1]

'Receptor'	Ligand	
	87.92.6	reovirus type 3
9BG5	$V_H\text{-}V_L > V_L$	$V_L = V_H\text{-}V_L$
Reo 3R	$V_H\text{-}V_L > V_L$	$V_L = V_H\text{-}V_L$

Ligand represents the substance competing with the peptide indicated. 'Receptor' indicates the material with which the peptides and the ligand interact. Reo3R = Reovirus type 3 receptor. $V_H\text{-}V_L = V_H\text{-}V_L$ peptide. $V_L = V_L$ peptide.
[1]The comparative strength of inhibition of the interactions noted by the peptides is indicated. See the text for full explanation.

CDR II and the HA3, seemed likely to be the relevant site for HA3 binding, and binding of its internal image as represented by 87.92.6.

Predicted Structure of the HA3 and 87.92.6 Receptor Interaction Sites

It was clear that the cell attachment site of the HA3 was both functionally and molecularly mimicked by the 87.92.6 light chain CDR II. It was reasoned that there might be a structural similarity between these two sites. This was supported by computer modeling of these regions utilizing the Chou and Fasman [61] algorithm. In both structures, a reverse turn was predicted to form at the sequence Tyr Ser Gly Ser. This sequence was identical in the V_L CDR II and in the HA3 (table 1).

It was reasoned that the structure of the V_L CDR II might be similar to the CDR IIs of other immunoglobulins. Several immunoglobulin structures have been determined from X-ray crystallographic data [2–4, 66]. Other antibody CDR IIs, with known structure, were searched for that shared amino acid sequence similarity with the putative cell attachment site identified on the HA3. The two best matches were the CDR IIs of REI (a human light chain dimer) and the heavy chain of NEWM (a human IgG$_1$) (table 3).

These CDR II structures were utilized according to the scheme shown in figure 5. The CDR II structures were isolated from the immunoglobulin structure. Where mismatches occurred, the appropriate amino acid side chains were substituted. Energy minimization calculations were then performed and the resultant structures analyzed.

Table 3. Amino acid sequences for the CDR II of REI (a human light chain dimer), the 87.92.6 heavy and light chain variable region CDR IIs (V_H and V_L respectively), and the heavy chain CDR II of NEWM (a human heavy chain) are shown aligned with the reovirus HA3 sequence: identities (●) and conservative substitutions (○) are indicated.

NEWM	Arg	Gly	Leu	Glu	Trp	Ilu	Gly	Tyr	Val	Phe	Tyr	His	Gly	Thr			
		●	●	●	●	●	●	○					○	○			
V_H	Gln	Gly	Leu	Glu	Trp	Ilu	Gly	Arg	Ilu	Asp	Pro	Ala	Asn	Gly			
	●	○	○		●	●	●	○									
Reo	Gln	Ser	Met	---	Trp	Ilu	Gly	Ilu	Val	Ser	Tyr	Ser	Gly	Ser	Gly	Leu	Asn
								○	○		●	●	●	●		●	○
V_L	Lys	Pro	Gly	Lys	Thr	Asn	Lys	Leu	Leu	Ilu	Tyr	Ser	Gly	Ser	Thr	Leu	Gln
	●	●	●				●	●	●	●	●			●	○	●	●
REI	Thr	Pro	Gly	Lys	Ala	Pro	Lys	Leu	Leu	Ilu	Tyr	Glu	Ala	Ser	Asn	Leu	Gln

A hybrid structure was also constructed, utilizing the amino-terminal half of the NEWM CDR II, and the carboxy-terminal half of REI. This structure was developed to optimize amino acid sequence similarity. As the NEWM sequence shared a greater degree of similarity with the V_H CDR II, we utilized this region in the hybrid (which consisted of the amino-terminal half of the structure). Similarly, the REI structure shared a greater degree of similarity with the V_L CDR II, so we utilized this region of the REI structure (including the carboxy-terminal half of the structure).

As can be seen from figure 5, the energy minimization calculations repositioned the side chains of the amino acid residues on the structures. In some cases, these calculations also resulted in folding of the amino- and carboxy-terminal ends of the structure. This is due to the way these structures are derived, being isolated from an immunoglobulin variable region. However, the reverse-turn regions were relatively unaffected.

Including the initial substituted models and the minimized structures, a total of six possible structures were developed. Two of the best models and the structures from which they were derived, are shown in figure 6. Figure 6a depicts a structure based primarily on the NEWM CDR II, while in figure 6b the structure of the REI CDR II was used. Although the conformation of the beta turn regions differ, we have shown that the side chain positions are similar for both structures [62, 63].

While these models are preliminary, they serve as a basis for further studies to more fully characterize the fine structure of this epitope. This sort

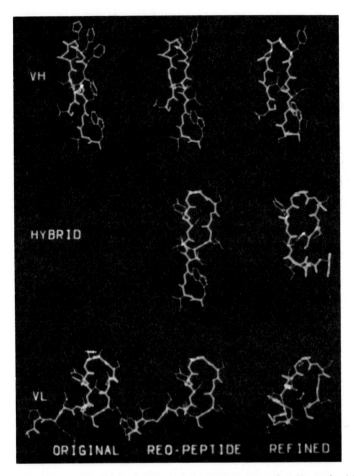

Fig. 5. Modeling of the reovirus type 3 cell attachment site. The excised CDR II loops of the NEWM heavy chain (top left) and the CDR II of REI (bottom left) are shown. These were modified by substituting amino acid side chains of the reovirus HA3 sequence (middle, top and bottom respectively). A hybrid structure, utilizing the regions with greatest amino acid sequence similarity, is also shown (middle, middle). Energy refined structures are shown on the right.

of mimicry, by internal image-bearing antibodies, should be a generally useful method for analyzing a variety of protein structures. When an antibody reproduces the biologic activity of another protein, this sort of analysis can be applied, and structures relevant for the activity of the protein and the internal image can be analyzed.

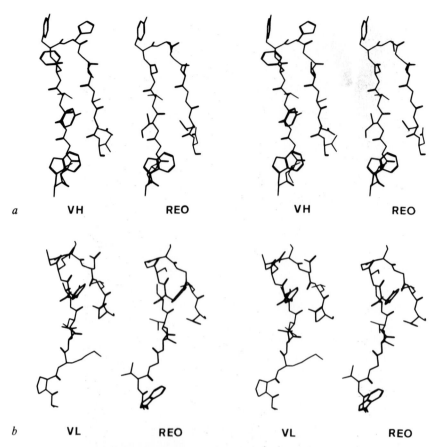

a   **VH**   **REO**   **VH**   **REO**

b   **VL**   **REO**   **VL**   **REO**

Fig. 6. Stereo drawings of the best models for the reovirus HA3 cell attachment site. The deduced structures are shown compared to the original CDR II loops from which they were derived. *a* The NEWM CDR II loop (V$_H$) is shown on the left and the deduced structure on the right (REO). *b* The REI CDR II loop (V$_L$) was utilized.

Regulatory Considerations

The functional nature of the internal image mimicry presented by 87.92.6 could have serious pathologic consequences. It has been demonstrated that when the reovirus HA3 bound to cell surface receptors, there was an immediate consequence on cellular metabolism. This included inhibition of DNA synthesis and cellular proliferation [36]. It was recently demonstrated that binding of 87.92.6 to the reovirus type 3 receptor induced similar changes [67]. The development of this kind of internal image antibody during an immune response would likely be detrimental to the host. Consequently, it would be advantageous for the host to have a mechanism by which the development of internal images could be regulated.

We have studied four independent mechanisms which implicated T cell regulation in this system [68, 69]. Cellular immunity to reovirus type 3 has been demonstrated to be strongly influenced by the hemagglutinin molecule [70, 73]. This included induction of helper (T_H), suppressor (T_s), cytotoxic (CTL), and delayed-type hypersensitivity (T_{DTH}) T cells. In at least 3 of these cases, cross-reactivity between the HA3 and 87.92.6 has been demonstrated [56, 57, 68, 69]. We will consider the potential regulatory role of each of these mechanisms separately.

T_H Regulation

It has been demonstrated that priming mice with reovirus type 3 induces T_H capable of responding to reovirus type 3, 87.92.6, and V_H peptide (derived from the 87.92.6 V_H CDR II) [68, 69]. This cross-reactivity is likely due to the sequence similarity shared by the HA3 and the V_H CDR II. T_H were demonstrated to proliferate and secrete lymphokines (interleukin 2) in response to V_H peptide, following reovirus type 3 priming. The development of these cross-reactive T_H, during the course of a primary immune response to reovirus type 3, might result in increased levels of internal image bearing antibodies.

This phenomenon suggests a positive regulation of internal image antibody development. This may have several consequences. Uncontrolled positive regulation, or inadequate suppression of this mechanism, could lead to high levels of internal image antibody production. This would include reovirus type 3 receptor-binding antibodies, and these immunoglobulins represent an autoreactive population (autoantibodies). This mechanism may be responsible for the development of some forms of antireceptor autoantibodies, and consequent pathologic changes.

Stimulation of internal image-bearing B cells, by cross-reactive T_H, might also have an effect on idiotype expression of the antireovirus response. Since 87.92.6 binds to anti-HA3 monoclonal 9BG5, a direct interaction between idiotype and internal image anti-idiotype could develop during the primary immune response. Note that the same cross-reactive T_H could stimulate both anti-HA3-bearing B cells (by virtue of their ability to bind, process and present HA3 determinants to T_H), and internal image-bearing B cells (by virtue of their presentation of processed internal image immuno-globulin determinants). Thus, both idiotypic and anti-idiotypic antibodies may develop concurrently. The interaction between these B cell subsets is likely to have an impact on the expression of both idiotype and internal anti-idiotype expression during the developing immune response. It is note-worthy that 9BG5 represents a dominant idiotype in the neutralizing anti-HA3 response in Balb/c mice. This set of interactions may be involved in the development of this idiotypic dominance.

T_s Regulation

The development of suppressor T cells in the response to reovirus type 3 has been previously demonstrated [70]. These T_s were largely specific for the hemagglutinin, and able to negatively regulate cellular immunity to reovirus. HA3-specific T_s were stimulated by reovirus type 3 bearing cells, and may be triggered by infected cells during the course of a primary immune response [70]. If these T_s recognize a similar determinant to the one described above, they could directly interact with internal image-bearing B cells, and negative-ly regulate their development. Alternatively, these T_s may interact with other T cell subsets involved in regulating the response. The net effect would be negative regulation of internal image-bearing B cells.

In addition, cross-reactive T_H induction of internal image-bearing anti-bodies may lead to the triggering of T_s. Several suppressor T cell circuits have been characterized. These demonstrate the participation of idiotype-anti-idiotype interactions in T_s regulation [74–76]. The development of T_s in response to either the HA3 or internal image-bearing antibodies, could feed back on the cross-reactive T_H, and act as a negative regulatory influence. T_s participation is likely to occur in the in vivo response to the HA3, and would impact on the nature and extent of the immune response.

Other T Cell Subsets

In addition to the above considerations, prior studies have demonstrated both CTL and T_{DTH} cross-reactive for the HA3 and 87.92.6 [56, 57]. Direct participation of either T_{DTH} or CTL would likely result in negative regulation of internal image antibody production.

Following reovirus type 3 stimulation, HA3-specific T_{DTH} and CTL develop [70, 71, 73]. Some of these T cells are likely to recognize internal image-bearing B cells. This recognition would trigger CTL to directly lyse these B cells, eliminating them and preventing further antibody production. T_{DTH} stimulated in a similar manner would elaborate cytokines which might act directly on B cells, or alternatively could promote T_{DTH} effector cell development with subsequent local nonspecific cytotoxicity [77]. In either case, the internal image-bearing B cells could be eliminated.

The existence of these regulatory mechanisms has been largely implicated from experimental studies. Whether these are active in vivo remains mainly speculative at this time. In addition, other regulatory mechanisms may affect internal image antibody production. The studies described above suggest mechanisms of internal image antibody regulation, all of which have experimental support, and which may be active in vivo. It is also unclear what regulatory events are operative to regulate these processes. However, it is apparent that the development of potentially pathologic antibodies is regulated by the immune system. Further studies may elucidate the role of the mechanisms described here, in the regulation of internal image antibody production.

References

1 Berzofsky, J.A.: Intrinsic and extrinsic factors in protein antigenic structure. Science *229:* 932–940 (1985).

2 Silverton, E.W.; Navia, M.A.; Davies, D.R.: Three-dimensional structure of an intact human immunoglobulin. Proc. natn. Acad. Sci. USA *74:* 5140–5144 (1977).

3 Edmundson, A.B.; Ely, K.R.; Abola, E.E.; Schiffer, M.; Panagiotopoulos, N.: Rotational allomerism and divergent evolution of domains in immunoglobulin light chains. Biochemistry *14:* 3953–3961 (1975).

4 Huber, R.; Deisenhofer, J.; Colman, P.M.; Matsushima, M.; Palm, W.: Crystallographic structure of an IgG molecule and an Fc fragment. Nature, Lond. *264:* 415–420 (1976).

5 Jerne, N.K.: Towards a network theory of the immune system. Ann. Immunol., Paris *125:* 373–389 (1974).

6 Gaulton, G.N.; Co, M.S.; Royer, H.-D.; Greene, M.I.: Anti-idiotypic antibodies as probes of cell surface receptors. Mol. cell. Biochem. *65:* 5–21 (1985).

7 Sege, K.; Peterson, P.A.: Anti-idiotypic antibodies against anti-vitamin A transporting protein react with prealbumin. Nature, Lond. *271:* 167–168 (1978).

8 Sege, K.; Peterson, P.A.: Use of anti-idiotypic antibodies as cell surface receptor probes. Proc. natn. Acad. Sci. USA *75:* 2443–2447 (1978).

9 Shechter, Y.; Maron, R.I.; Elias, D.; Cohen, I.R.: Autoantibodies to insulin reeceptor spontaneously develop as anti-idiotypes in mice immunized with insulin. Science *216:* 542–545 (1982).

10 Shechter, Y.; Elias, D.; Maron, R.; Cohen, I.R.: Mouse antibodies to the insulin

receptor developing spontaneously as anti-idiotypes. I. Characterization of the antibodies. J. biol. Chem. *259:* 6411–6415 (1984).

11 Homcy, C.J.; Rockson, S.G.; Haber, E.: An anti-idiotypic antibody that recognizes the beta adrenergic receptor. J. clin. Invest. *69:* 1147–1154 (1982).

12 Schreiber, A.B.; Conrand, P.O.; André, C.; Vray, B.; Strosberg, A.D.: Anti-alperolol anti-idiotypic antibodies bind to beta-adrenergic receptors and modulate catecholanite-sensitive adenylate cyclase. Proc. natn. Acad. Sci. USA *77:* 7385–7389 (1980).

13 Marasco, W.A.; Becker, E.L.: Anti-idiotype as antibody against the formyl peptide chemotaxis receptor of the neutrophil. J. Immun. *128:* 963–968 (1982).

14 Lambris, J.D.; Ross, G.D.: Characterization of the lymphocyte membrane receptor for factor H (beta-1-H globulin) with an antibody to anti-factor H idiotype. J. exp. Med. *155:* 1400–1411 (1982).

15 Erlanger, B.F.; Cleveland, W.L.; Wassermann, N.H.; Ku, H.H.; Hill, B.L.; Sarangarajan, R.; Rajagopalan, R.; Cayanis, E.; Edelman, I.S.; Penn, A.S.: Auto-anti-idiotype. A basis for autoimmunity and a strategy for anti-receptor antibodies. Immunol. Rev. *94:* 23–27 (1986).

16 Nepom, J.T.; Tarideau, M.; Epstein, R.L.; Weiner, H.L.; Gentsch, J.; Fields, B.N.; Greene, M.I.: Virus binding receptors. Similarities to immune receptors as determined by anti-idiotypic antibodies. Immunol. Res. *1:* 255–261 (1982).

17 Co, M.S.; Gaulton, G.N.; Fields, B.N.; Greene, M.I.: Isolation and biochemical characterization of the mammalian reovirus type 3 cell-surface receptor. Proc. natn. Acad. Sci. USA *82:* 1494–1498 (1985).

18 Noseworthy, J.H.; Fields, B.N.; Dichter, M.A.; Sobotka, C.; Pizer, E.; Perry, L.L.; Nepom, J.T.; Greene, M.I.: Cell receptors for the mammalian reovirus. I. Syngeneic monoclonal anti-idiotypic antibody identifies a cell surface receptor for reovirus. J. Immun. *131:* 2533–2538 (1983).

19 Kauffman, R.S.; Noseworthy, J.H.; Nepom, J.T.; Finberg, R.; Fields, B.N.; Greene, M.I.: Cell receptors for mammalian reovirus. II. Monoclonal anti-idiotypic antibody blocks viral binding to cells. J. Immun. *131:* 2539–2541 (1983).

20 Thorbecke, G.J.; Siskind, G.W.: Auto-anti-idiotype production during response to antigen; in Greene, Nissonoff, The biology of idiotypes, pp. 417–434. (Plenum Press, New York 1984).

21 Joklik, W.K.: The reoviridae (Plenum Press, New York 1983).

22 Rosen, L.: Serologic graphing of reoviruses by hemagglutination inhibition. Am. J. Hyg. *71:* 242–249 (1960).

23 Rubin, D.H.; Fields, B.N.: Molecular basis of reovirus virulence. Role of the M2 gene. J. exp. Med. *152:* 853–868 (1980).

24 Weiner, H.L.; Powers, M.L.; Fields, B.N.: Absolute linkage of virulence and central nervous system cell tropism of reovioruses to viral hemagglutinin. J. infect. Dis. *141:* 609–619 (1980).

25 Weiner, H.L.; Drayna, D.; Avrill, D.R., Jr.; Fields, B.N.: Molecular basis of reovirus virulence. Role of the S1 gene. Proc. natn. Acad. Sci. USA *74:* 5744–5748 (1977).

26 Kaye, K.M.; Spriggs, D.R.; Bassel-Duby, R.; Fields, B.N.; Tyler, K.L.: Genetic basis for altered pathogenesis of an immune-selected antigenic variant of reovirus type 3 (Dearing). J. Virol. *59:* 90–97 (1986).

27 Greene, M.I.: Unpublished observations.

28 Wolf, J.L.; Rubin, D.H.; Finberg, R.; Kauffman, R.S.; Sharpe, A.H.; Trier, J.S.;
    Fields, B.N.: Intestinal M cells. A pathway for entry of reovirus into the host. Science
    212: 471–472 (1981).
29 Kilham, L.; Margolis, G.: Hydrocephalus in hamsters, ferrets, rats and mice follow-
    ing inoculations with reovirus type I. I. Virologic studies. Lab. Invest. *2:* 183–188
    (1969).
30 Raine, C.S.; Fields, B.N.: Reovirus type 3 encephalitis. A virologic and ultrastruc-
    tural study. J. Neuropath. exp. Neurol. *32:* 19–33 (1973).
31 Maratos-Flier, E.; Goodman, M.J.; Murray, A.H.; Kahn, C.R.: Ammonium inhibits
    processing and cytotoxicity of reovirus, a nonenveloped virus. J. clin. Invest. *78:*
    1003–1007 (1986).
32 Lee, P.W.K.; Hayes, E.C.; Joklik, W.K.: Characterization of anti-reovirus immuno-
    globulins secreted by cloned hybridoma cell lines. Virology *108:* 134–146 (1981).
33 Epstein, R.L.; Powers, M.L.; Rogart, R.B.; Weiner, H.L.: Binding of ^{125}I-labeled
    reovirus to cells surface receptors. Virology *133:* 46–55 (1984).
34 Weiner, D.B.; Girard, K.; Williams, W.V.; McPhillips, T.; Rubin, D.H.: Reovirus
    type 1 and 3 differ in their binding to intestinal epithelial cells. Microbial Pathogen.
    5: 29–40 (1988).
35 Gonatas, P.J.; Tamm, I.: Macromolecular synthesis in reovirus-infected cells. Bio-
    chim. biophys. Acta *72:* 651–653 (1963).
36 Sharpe, A.H.; Fields, B.N.: Reovirus inhibition of cellular DNA synthesis. Role of
    the S1 gene. J. Virol. *38:* 389–392 (1981).
37 Burstin, S.J.; Spriggs, D.R.; Fields, B.N.: Evidence for functional domains on the
    reovirus type 3 hemagglutinin. Virology *117:* 146–155 (1982).
38 Spriggs, D.R.; Kaye, K.; Fields, B.N.: Topological analysis of the reovirus type 3
    hemagglutinin. Virology *127:* 220–224 (1983).
39 Lee, P.W.K.; Hayes, E.C.; Joklik, W.K.: Protein σ 1 is the reovirus cell attachment
    protein. Virology *108:* 156–163 (1981).
40 Nepom, J.J.; Weiner, H.L.; Dichter, M.A.; Tardrieu, M.; Spriggs, D.R.; Gramm,
    C.F.; Powers, M.L.; Fields, B.W.; Greene, M.I.: Identification of a hemagglutinin-
    specific idiotype associated with reovirus recognition shared by lymphoid and neural
    cells. J. exp. Med. *155:* 155–167 (1982).
41 Gaulton, G.; Co, M.S.; Greene, M.I.: Anti-idiotypic antibody identifies the cellular
    receptor of reovirus type 3. J. cell. Biochem. *28:* 69–78 (1985).
42 Co, M.S.; Gaulton, G.N.; Tominager, A.; Homcy, C.J.; Fields, B.N.; Greene, M.I.:
    Structural similarities between the mammalian B-adrenergic receptor and reovirus
    type 3 receptors. Proc. natn. Acad. Sci. USA *82:* 5315–5318 (1985).
43 Liu, J.; Co, M.S.; Greene, M.I.: Reovirus type 3 and [I^{125}]-iodocyanopindolol bind to
    distinct domains of the reovirus receptor. Immunol. Res. *7:* 233–238 (1988).
44 Dixon, R.A.F.; Koblinka, B.K.; Strader, D.J.; Benovic, J.L.; Dohlman, H.G.; Frielle,
    T.; Bolanowski, M.A.; Bennett, C.D.; Rands, E.; Diehl, R.E.; Mumford, R.A.; Slater,
    E.E.; Sigal, I.S.; Caron, M.G.; Lefkowitz, R.J.; Strader, C.D.: Cloning of the gene and
    cDNA for the mammalian B-adrenergic receptor and homology with rhodopsin.
    Nature, Lond. *321:* 75–79 (1986).
46 Frielle, T.; Collins, S.; Daniel, K.W.; Caron, M.G.; Lefkowitz, R.J.; Koblika, B.K.:
    Cloning of the cDNA for the human β_1-adrenergic receptor. Proc. natn. Acad. Sci.
    USA *84:* 7920–7924 (1987).
47 Kubo, T.; Fukuda, K.; Mikami, A.; Maeda, A.; Takahashi, H.; Mishina, M.; Haga, T.;

Haga, K.; Ichiyama, A.; Kangawa,, K.; et al.: Cloning, sequencing and expression of complementary DNA encoding the muscarinic acetylcholine receptor. Nature, Lond. *323:* 411–416 (1986)

48 Ovchinnikov, Y.A.: Rhodopsin and bacteriorhodopsin. Structure-function relationships. FEBS Lett.*148:* 179–191 (1982).

49 Stryer, L.: Cyclic GMP cascade of vision. A. Rev. Neurosci. *9:* 87–119 (1986).

50 Khorana, H.G.; Gerber, G.E.; Herlihy, W.C.; Gray, C.P.; Anderegg, R.J.; Nihei, K.; Biemann, K.: Amino acid sequence of bacteriorhodopsin. Proc. natn. Acad. Sci. USA *76:* 5046–5050 (1979).

51 Nathans, J.; Thomas, D.; Hogness, D.S.: Molecular genetics of human color vision: the genes encoding blue, green and red pigments, Science *232:* 193–202 (1986).

52 Burkholder, A.C.; Hartwell, L.H.: The yeast alpha-factor receptor: structural properties deduced from the sequence of the STE2 gene. Nucl. Acids Res. *13:* 8463–8475 (1985).

53 Miyajima, I.; Nakafuku, M.; Nakayama, N.; Brenner, C.; Miyajima, A.; Kaibuchi, K.; Arai, K.; Kaziro, Y.; Matsumoto, K.: GPA1, a haploid-specific essential gene, encodes a yeast homolog of mammalian G protein which may be involved in mating factor signal transduction. Cell *50:* 1011 1019 (1987),

54 Young, D.; Waitches, G.; Birchmeier, C.; Fasano, O.; Wigler, M.: Isolation and characterization of a new cellular oncogene encoding a protein with multiple potential transmembrane domains. Cell *45:* 711–719 (1986).

55 Chin, D.J.; Gil, G.; Russel, D.W.; Liscum, L.; Luskey, K.L.; Basu, S.K.; Okayama, H.; Berg, P.; Goldstein, J.L.; Brown, M.S.: Nucleotide sequence of 3-hydroxy-3-methyl-glutaryl coenzyme A reductase, a glycoprotein of endoplasmic reticulum. Nature, Lond. *308:* 613–617 (1984).

56 Sharpe, A.H.; Gaulton, G.N.; McDade, K.K.; Fields, B.N.; Greene, M.I.: Syngeneic monoclonal antiidiotype can induce cellular immunity to reovirus. J. exp. Med. *160:* 195–205 (1984).

57 Sharpe. A.H.; Gaulton, G.N.; Ertl, H.C.J.; Finberg, R.W.; McDade, K.K.; Fields, B.N.; Greene, M.I.: Cell receptors for the mammalian reovirus IV. Reovirus-specific cytolytic T cell lines that have idiotypic receptors recognize anti-idiotypic B cell hybridomas. J. Immun. *134:* 2702–2706 (1985).

58 Gaulton, G.N.; Sharpe, A.H.; Chang, D.W.; Fields, B.N.; Greene, M.I.: Syngeneic monoclonal internal image anti-idiotypes as prophylactic vaccines. J. Immun. *137:* 2930–2936 (1986).

59 Bruck, C.; Co, M.S.; Slaoui, M.; Gaulton, G.N.; Smith, T.; Fields, B.N.; Mullins, J.I.; Greene, M.I.: Nucleic acid sequence of an internal image-bearing monoclonal anti-idiotype and its comparison to the sequence of the external antigen. Proc. natn. Acad. Sci. USA *83:* 6578–6582 (1986).

60 Bassel-Duby, R.; Jayasuriya, A.; Chatterjee, D.; Sonenberg, N.; Maizel, J.V., Jr.; Fields, B.N.: Sequence of reovirus hemagglutinin predicts a coiled-coil structure. Nature, Lond. *315:* 421–423 (1985).

61 Chou, P.Y.; Fasman, G.D.: Prediction of protein conformation. Biochemistry *13:* 222–245 (1974).

62 Williams, W.V.; Guy, H.R.; Rubin, D.H.; Robey, F.; Myers, J.N.; Kieber-Emmons, T.; Weiner, D.B.; Greene, M.I.: Sequence of the cell-attachment site of reovirus type and its anti-idiotype/antireceptor antibody: Modeling of their three-dimensional structures. Proc. natn. Acad. Sci. USA *85:* 6488–6492 (1988).

63 Williams, W.V.; Guy, H.R.; Weiner, D.; Rubin, D.; Greene, M.I.: Structure of the neutralizing epitope of the reovirus type 3 hemagglutinin; in Vaccines 88, pp. 25 –28 (Cold Spring Harbor Press, New York, 1988).

64 Williams, W.V.; Guy, H.R.; Greene, M.I.: Three dimensional structure of a functional internal image. Viral Immunol. (in press, 1989).

65 Williams, W.V.; Weiner, D.B.; Rubin, D.H.; Guy, H.R.; Greene, M.I.: Determination of the neutralizing/cell attachment epitope of reovirus type 3. Technological Advances in Vaccine Development, pp. 577–586 (Alan R. Liss Inc. NY 1988).

66 Bernstein, F.C.; Koetzle, T.F.; Williams, G.J.; Meyer, E.F., Jr.; Brice, M.D.; Rodgers, J.R.; Kennard, O.; Shimanouchi, T.; Tasumi, M.: The protein data bank: a computer-based archival file for macromolecular structures. Eur. J. Biochem. 80: 319–324 (1977).

67 Gaulton, G.N.; Greene, M.I.: Inhibition of cellular DNA synthesis by reovirus occurs through a receptor-linked signalling pathway which is mimicked by anti-receptor antibody. J. exp. Med. 169: 197–212 (1989).

68 Williams, W.V.; London, S.L.; Rubin, D.H.; Wadsworth, S.; Weiner, D.B.; Berzofsky, J.; Greene, M.I.: Immune response to a molecularly defined internal image idiotope. J. Immunol. (in press).

69 Williams, W.V.; Weiner, D.B.; Rubin, D.H.; Greene, M.I.: Antigenic structure of the neutralizing epitope of reovirus type 3. Immun. Allergy Clins. N. Am. 8: 169–172 (1988).

70 Greene, M.I.; Weiner, H.L.: Delayed hypersensitivity in mice infected with reovirus. II. Induction of tolerance and suppressor T cells to viral specific gene products. J. Immun. 124: 282–287 (1980).

71 Weiner, H.L.; Greene, M.I.; Fields, B.N.: Delayed type hypersensitivity in mice infected with reovirus. I. Identification of host and viral gene products responsible for the immune response. J. Immun. 125: 278–282 (1980).

72 Matsuzaki, N.; Hinshaw, V.S.; Fields, B.N.; Greene, M.I.: Cell receptors for the mammalian reovirus. Reovirus-specific T-cell hybridomas can become persistently infected and undergo autoimmune stimulation. J. Virol. 60: 259–266 (1986).

73 Finberg, R.; Spriggs, D.R.; Fields, B.N.: Host immune response to reovirus: CTL recognize the major neutralization domain of the viral hemagglutinin. J. Immun. 129: 2235–2238 (1982).

74 Sy, M.-S.; Dietz, M.H.; Germain, R.N.: Antigen and receptor driven regulatory mechanisms. IV. Idiotype bearing I-J$^+$ suppressor T cell factors induce second-order suppressor T cells which express anti-idiotypic receptors. J. exp. Med. 151: 1183–1195 (1980).

75 Sy, M.-S.; Nisonoff, A.; Germain, R.N.; Benacerraf, B.; Greene, M.I.: Antigen and receptor-driven regulatory mechanisms. Suppression of idiotype-negative-p-azobenzenearsonate specific T cells results from the interaction of an anti-idiotypic second order T suppressor cell with a cross-reactive-idiotype positive p-azobenzenearsonate-primed T cell target. J. exp. Med. 133: 1415–1425 (1981).

76 Sy, M.-S.; Brown, A.; Bach, B.A.; Benacerraf, B.; Gottlieb, P.D.; Nisonoff, A.; Greene, M.I.: Genetic and serological analysis of the expression of crossreactive idiotypic determinants on anti-p-azobenzenearsonate antibodies and p-azobenzene-arsonate-specific suppressor T cell factors. Proc. natn. Acad. Sci. USA 78: 1143–1147 (1981).

77 Greene, M.I.; Schatten, S.; Bromberg, J.S.: Delayed hypersensitivity; in Paul, Fundamental immunology, pp. 685–696 (Raven Press, New York 1984).
78 Wasserman, R.L.; Capa, J.D.: Immunoglobulins; in Horowitz, Pigman, The glycoproteins, pp. 323–348 (Academic Press, New York 1977).
79 Kabat, E.A.; Wu, T.T.; Reid-Miller, M.; Perry, H.M.; Gottesman, K.S.: Sequences of proteins of immunologic interest; 4th ed. (US Department of Health & Human Services, Public Health Service, National Institutes of Health, Bethesda 1987).

William V. Williams, MD, Department of Pathology and Laboratory Medicine, University of Pennsylvania School of Medicine, Room 252, John Morgan Building, 36th Street and Hamilton Walk, Philadelphia, PA 19104 (USA)

Subject Index